# Acute
# Heart Failure

Putting the Puzzle of Pathophysiology
and Evidence Together in Daily Practice

Wolfgang Krüger and Andrew Ludman

Birkhäuser
Basel · Boston · Berlin

Dr. Wolfgang Krüger
Queen Elizabeth Hospital
Stadium Road
London SE18 4QH
United Kingdom

Dr. Andrew J. Ludman
Royal Free & University College
Medical School
Hatter Cardiovascular Institute
Division of Medicine
67 Chenies Mews
London WClE 6HX
United Kingdom

Library of Congress Control Number: 2009923284

Bibliographic information published by Die Deutsche Bibliothek:
Die Deutsche Bibliothek lists this publication in the Deutsche Nationalbibliografie;
detailed bibliographic data is available in the Internet at <http://dnb.ddb.de>

ISBN  978-3-0346-0021-7   Birkhäuser Verlag AG, Basel · Boston · Berlin

© 2009 Birkhäuser Verlag AG
Basel · Boston · Berlin
P.O. Box 133, CH-4010 Basel, Switzerland
Part of Springer Science+Business Media
Printed on acid-free paper produced from chlorine-free pulp. TCF ∞
Cover Design: B. Blankenburg and K. Tüchert, Birkhäuser, Basel
Cover Illustration: Human Heart: © Zygote Media Group Inc. / Diagram: see page 25,
© Massachusetts Medical Society. All rights reserved
Typeset: HD Ecker: TeXtservices, Bonn
Graphics: Modified by K. Uplegger, Birkhäuser, Basel
Printed in Germany

ISBN 978-3-0346-0021-7                          e-ISBN 978-3-0346-0022-4
9 8 7 6 5 4 3 2 1                               www.birkhauser.ch

# Contents

# Foreword

Heart failure is one of the leading causes of morbidity and mortality in Europe and the United States of America. The incidence within the European population is estimated to range between 0.4 to 2.0%, and in the USA approximately one million people per year are admitted to hospital suffering from heart failure.

Despite the best efforts of health care professionals, the prognosis of heart failure remains poor with a 60–90 day mortality of approximately 10%. Recently published analyses of clinical practice have revealed a 'gap' between the evidence base for the management of acute heart failure and the reality of day to day medical care.

With this book we aim to bridge the 'evidence gap' and provide a highly evidenced based guide to the pathophysiology and management of acute heart failure syndromes. Chapter 1 guides the reader through a broad background of pathophysiological concepts and underlying theories of the development and management of acute heart failure. In chapter 2, the classification of acute heart failure is addressed and how this aids management. Chapter 3 deals with the difficult scenario of cardiogenic shock and how an evidenced based approach may help current management and point to future potential therapeutic strategies. Chapters 4 and 5 deal with the less common but increasingly important areas of acute right heart failure and heart failure with normal ejection fraction. These conditions have previously been neglected but are recognised to contribute significantly to the morbidity and mortality associated with acute heart failure and as such these chapters are essential reading.

This book will appeal to the wide variety of health care professionals, from a broad cross section of specialties, who come in to contact with this complex group of patients. Using a heavily referenced approach we aim to equip trainees, junior and senior practitioners with the latest theories on the pathophysiology behind, and the management of, acute heart failure. Older theories are recapped and appraised with the latest data, and new theories, yet to be established in main stream clinical care, are introduced. By using diagrams to illustrate complex issues and deriving some concepts from first principles the reader will be able to retain and pass on to colleagues the pathophysiological principles which should underpin a thorough understanding of this heterogeneous disease.

Above all, we hope the reader will enjoy this text as we aim to promote interest, discussion and further exploration of this area. There is still a long way to go in improving the outcomes of patients with acute heart failure.

Dr Wolfgang Krüger
Dr Andrew Ludman
January 2009

# Chapter 1

## Cardiac physiology of acute heart failure syndromes

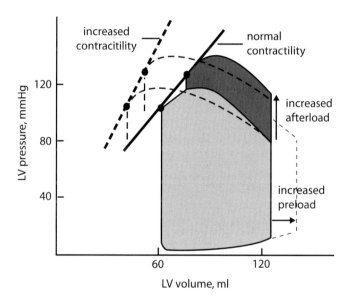

Adapted from Mohrman, DE and Heller, LJ, *Cardiovascular Physiology*, 4th ed. McGraw-Hill Comp., 1997, chapter 4, p. 69.

## 1.1    Cardiac performance

Cardiac performance depends on a wide variety of factors, of which preload, afterload, heart rate, and contractility are the best recognised. However, other factors play important roles but are less acknowledged. The diastolic ventricular interaction (DVI) and its impact on preload, the preload recruitable stroke-work, ventriculo-arterial coupling and other vascular and ventricular properties, through their interaction at end-systole, all have significant influence on cardiac performance.

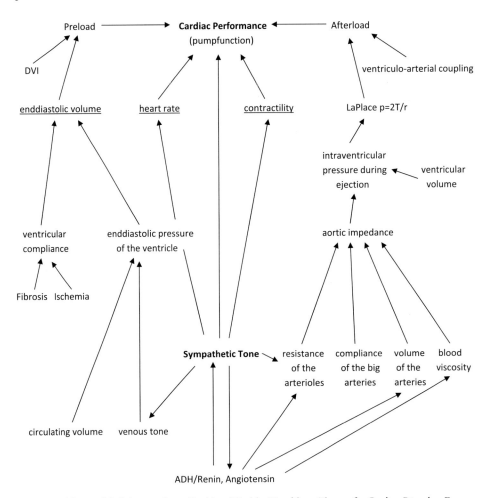

**Figure 1.1** The modified diagram from Gould and Reddy, *Vasodilator Therapy for Cardiac Disorders*, Futura, Mount Kisco, New York, 1979, pp. 1–6, illustrates the complex interplay of factors affecting cardiac performance.

## 1.2 The fundamental equation of the circulation

$$MAP = CO \times SVR \text{ (Pressure = Flow} \times \text{Resistance) [1, 2]}$$

The fundamental equation of the circulatory system expresses the basic function of the heart: to generate flow **and** pressure in order to ensure appropriate perfusion of the body [3, 4].

The systemic peripheral resistance, difficult to determine directly in practice, can be calculated by using the measurable parameters of MAP and CO. However the SVR is **not** determined by them, **SVR and CO are independent, the MAP is the dependent variable** [5].

Poiseuille's law offers three ways to change blood pressure [6, 7]:
- alter flow,
- alter resistance,
- alter both.

Thus, increased blood flow and/or an increased ratio of resistance/blood flow (SVR/CO) can alter the MAP [8]. If CO and SVR change **reciprocally and proportionately,** only then will the MAP be unchanged. If CO increases but with a reduction of SVR due to peripheral vasodilatation, MAP will increase if the increase in CO is proportionally higher than the reduction of SVR. In the case of **volume loading, increasing CO will lead to an increase in MAP if SVR remains unchanged** [5].

Kumar showed that volume loading in **healthy hearts** increases contractility, stroke work, systolic blood pressure, **and MAP** [9]. However, in the heart with compromised contractility, blood pressure might not increase. Michard [10] showed that the increase in SV (flow) depends critically on the contractile abilities of the heart (see figure 1.4). Thus, if volume loading does not lead to an increase in SV, we should be suspicious of significant heart failure. Furthermore, we should keep in mind that, in heart failure syndromes, the **LV afterload** is the decisive determinant of cardiac performance [11–15]. Therefore, a reduction in afterload by vasodilators is the treatment of choice [16, 17].

As a rule, in **daily clinical practice** in acute heart failure when **lowering peripheral resistance**, the LV end-systolic wall stress will be reduced and the **SV will increase,** but the MAP will be maintained or will even increase [18–20]. If, under these conditions, the MAP does not increase or at least cannot be maintained, the following circumstances have to be considered:

- severe mitral regurgitation [21–25],
- inappropriate filling of the LV due to **DVI** [26–29],
- ventriculo-arterial coupling mismatch [30–32],
- inadequate intravascular volume (relative hypovolaemia) [33–35] – (seldom).

## 1.3    Preload

### a)    Definition

Preload is defined by Braunwald and Ross [36] as "**the force acting to stretch the left ventricular muscle fibres at the end of diastole** and **determining the resting length of the sarcomeres**".

Returning venous blood fills the ventricle, exerting force on the heart muscle, stretching the myofibrils [36] and is one of the main determinants of cardiac performance [37–39].

The end-diastolic ventricular volume, or preload, is well reflected by the end-diastolic wall stress (**preload ~ end-diastolic wall stress**) [40].

### b)    The Frank–Starling mechanism

**Transmural** LVEDP accurately reflects the effective distending pressure responsible for the length of myocardial fibres [41].

Otto Frank [42] and Ernest Starling [43] obtained a relationship between the end-diastolic fibre length and the force of contraction:

**With increasing fibre length the force of contraction increases** and thus the **LV or RV stroke volume (SV)** [42, 43] **increases** or, more accurately, the stroke work (SW) increases:

$$LV\text{-}SW = SV \times (LVESP - LVEDP) \text{ [30, 44]}$$

The diastolic ventricular filling is limited by the acutely non-distensible pericardium constraining the filling ventricles and by the cytoskeleton [45–47], thus preventing the ventricles from fluid overload [48, 49] (physiological protective mechanism) as well as from pathological dilatation [45].

With an increase in resting fibre length the velocity of fibre muscle shortening increases as well [50].

Frank [42] established a linear relationship between the left ventricular **end-diastolic volume** (LVEDV) as a correlate of the fibre length and the **force of ventricular contraction** [36, 42, 43, 48].

LV-SV correlates well with LVEDV: **SV ~ LVEDV** [51].

Starling [43] reported an increase in the **contraction force** with increasing atrial **pressures**.

Starling's result is similar to that described by Frank, as long as the increase in LVEDP represents a **proportional** increase in LVEDV (linear relationship between LVEDP and LVEDV). This is true in most healthy persons as long as the LVEDP remains within normal ranges, but in the case of high LV filling pressures and in certain pathological circumstances the rise in LVEDP is often disproportionately high in comparison to the increase in LVEDV [26, 27, 52–55].

The LVEDP may even rise without any increase in LV filling volume, producing no increase in preload, which is essential to recruit a higher SV [26, 30, 46]. Therefore, although the LVEDP rises, there may be no adequate increase in SV; in fact, there may even be a fall corresponding with the 'descending limb' of the Starling curve [30, 41, 43, 56]. This descending limb described by Starling is, however, an artefact of his experimental conditions.

When using the **effective distending pressure** rather than the intra-cavitary pressure the relation between fibre stretch and force of contraction is described adequately and corresponds to Frank's findings and the statement:

The effective distending pressure or '**transmural**' **LVEDP** is the intracavitary **LVEDP** (commonly just called LVEDP) **minus** the **surrounding pressure(s)** [41].

Katz, in 1965, already assumed that intracavitary and transmural end-diastolic left ventricular pressures were only equal when the pressure surrounding the left ventricular heart muscle was negligible [41]. Otherwise the external pressure must be subtracted from the intracavitary LVEDP to calculate the effective distending or transmural pressure.

$$\text{Transmural LVEDP} = \text{LVEDP} - \text{surrounding pressure [41]}$$

Usually, the surrounding pressure has contributions of one-third by the RVEDP and two-thirds by the pericardial pressure [57, 58]:

$$\text{Transmural LVEDP} = \text{intracavitary LVEDP} - (2/3 \text{ pericardial pressure} + 1/3 \text{ RVEDP})$$

Under normal conditions, RAP and pericardial pressure (PP) are nearly equal [59–61] and further changes in pericardial pressure are very closely reflected by RA pressure changes [59, 62, 63].

The close relation between changes in RA pressure and pericardial pressures allows us to give a reasonable estimate of transmural pressure by subtracting RAP from pulmonary capillary wedge pressure (PCWP) [26, 59, 62]:

$$\text{Transmural LVEDP} = \text{PCWP} - \text{RAP} \approx \text{PCWP} - \text{CVP}$$

with CVP reflecting the 'surrounding pressure' [26, 59, 62, 64–66].

There is substantial evidence that PCWP reflects LVEDP [67–69]. CVP is measured where the vena cava leads into the right atrium [64] and, as such, equals the RAP [64–66]. Due to the very close relations between RAP and PP (r = 0.95, p < 0.005) [71] and RAP and changes in PP [59, 62, 63] respectively, CVP is a good estimate of PP [59–66, 71] in daily practice. Furthermore, both, CVP and RAP reflect the RVEDP [49, 65, 66, 70, 71], RV-failure will cause a rise in CVP [64].

In healthy persons the surrounding pressure is low (nearly zero) and an increase in preload will increase the LVEDP more than the surrounding pressure [26, 45]. Hence, the transmural LVEDP will rise along with LVEDV [26, 48, 72], increasing the preload recruitable stroke volume (work) and thus SV, as described by Frank and Starling.

In conditions where the surrounding pressure rises substantially, external constraint increases more than LVEDP [26, 27, 52–55, 73–75]. Transmural LVEDP and intracavitary LVEDP will differ considerably and will change in opposite directions with a fall in transmural LVEDP, lowering the preload and, consequently, the preload recruitable stroke volume (work) will decrease.

The intraventricular pressures (intracavitary LVEDP and RVEDP) are influenced by:

- LV-compliance [76],
- alteration in lung anatomy and physiology-inducing changes in the intrathoracic pressure [52] and the pressures in the pulmonary circulation [77],
- intra-abdominal pressure [78].

The LV compliance describes the diastolic properties of the heart muscle and can be depicted by the relation between LVEDP and LVEDV [57, 79] (relation between pressure and volume).

With this in mind, the discrepancies between transmural LVEDP and intracavitary LVEDP can be related, at least partly, to the ventricular compliance [80].

The ventricular compliance varies almost continuously in the critically ill, producing changes in the intracavitary LVED<u>P</u> but without any corresponding change in LVED<u>V</u> [76, 81, 82]. Kumar [83], however, established evidence that continuous change in the ventricular compliance is a physiological phenomenon present in healthy persons as well as in those who are unwell.

In heart failure, the compliance of the LV is almost always reduced [56]; hence, increases in filling volumes cause a higher rise in LVEDP compared to a healthy heart.

The compliance is determined by factors such as muscle mass, tissue composition, elastic properties, ventricular interactions and extramyocardial conditions including pericardial structure and intrathoracic properties [84–88].

Raised intrathoracic pressure due to pneumonia, ARDS, pulmonary oedema, etc., as well as raised intra-abdominal pressure will increase constraint, in particular on the thin-walled RV, affecting the RVEDP and PP more than the LVEDP [52].

Furthermore, the higher the LVEDP the greater the amount of external force acting on the LV, thus impeding the LV-filling, the preload, and preload recruitable SV (SW) [27, 28].

Examples of situations which alter the surrounding pressures or produce significant external pericardial constraint are:

- increased lung water due to congestive HF [89],
- mechanical ventilation and PEEP: Both induce a rise in intrathoracic pressure (surrounding pressure) and an increase in RV-afterload [90]. The normally low RVEDP and PP will rise markedly in case of mechanical positive pressure ventilation and/or PEEP application, pneumonia, ARDS, etc., and so contribute essentially to an increase in the surrounding pressure [62];
- In heart failure patients we expect a marked external constraint to be present in the majority of patients, compromising LV-filling and becoming significant if LVEDP > 10(12)–15 mm Hg [27, 28, 91]. Physiological external constraint, mainly due to PP, contributes up to 30–40% of the LVEDP [28]. In heart failure the contribution to LVEDP by the external constraint is as high as 50–80% [26];
- acute pulmonary embolism: ↑ RVEDP and thus ↑ in PP [52], hence a rise in the surrounding pressure inducing no change [52] or even ↓ in the transmural LVEDP [30].

In the case of external constraint, LVEDP markedly overestimates effective distending pressure [46].

Changes in opposite directions (transmural LVEDP ↓ and intracavitary LVEDP ↑) are explainable now, and **only** an **increase in transmural LVEDP is consistent with an increase in LVEDV** and vice versa [26, 30, 46].

Numerous publications have established that haemodynamic monitoring by PA-catheterisation measuring intracavitary (filling-) pressures fails to be an accurate guide of the preload because filling pressures do not adequately reflect the myocardial fibre length at end-diastole and, hence, the LVEDV [42, 92–94]. If the transmural pressure is used instead, then changes in the preload are accurately reflected [41].

However, the filling pressures are still one of the most important components in assessment and treatment decision-making processes in heart failure. The heart always tries to generate an adequate CO on the lowest possible LVEDP [80, 92, 95]. In heart failure patients, a therapeutic reduction of the LVEDP is correlated with improved outcome [96, 97]; hence, unloading the left ventricle and reducing the LVEDP is the therapeutic maxim that adheres to the physiology/pathophysiology of the situation [26, 27, 42, 43, 56] and improves outcome [16, 17, 27, 96]. Thus, we might do much better in our patients with severe heart failure and cardiogenic shock using the transmural LVEDP to make our therapeutic decisions.

There is, of course, a physiological optimum and maximum of fibre distension and concomitant force development (see Figure 1.2) [98].

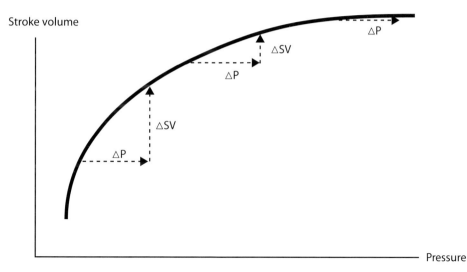

**Figure 1.2** Δp: Change in pressure; ΔSV: Change in SV; with increasing transmural pressure and thus preload, the recruited SV becomes less (modified from Michard [10]).

Furthermore, in the situation of (acute) heart failure the **Frank–Starling mechanism is markedly diminished** [56] and thus, in the failing heart, an increase in fibre stretch (ventricular filling) is not accompanied by the same increase in the force of contraction as in healthy persons [99].

In the **failing heart** the SV depends **substantially** on the contractility [10, 82, 100, 101] **and** the **afterload** [3, 13, 51, 102, 103].

## c)      Venous return and CVP in daily practice

SV is determined by venous return (responsible for the preload) and cardiac performance (contractility, afterload and heart rate) [37–39].

Guyton [38] evaluated the relationship between total cardiac function (contractility and total peripheral resistance) and venous return:

"The actual cardiac output changes with changes in cardiac function (CF), but with changes in venous return as well".

He plotted the relationships (total cardiac function and venous return) on **one** graph (see Figure 1.3) [38].

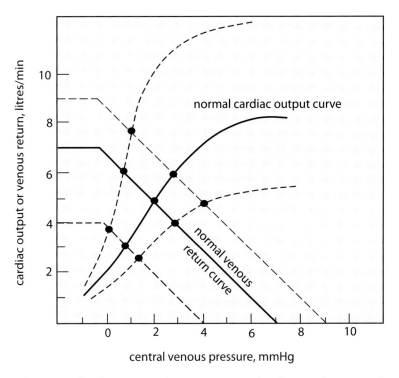

**Figure 1.3** The upper cardiac function curve depicts a supra-normal performance (i.e. ↑ sympathetic tone) while the lower curve represents the situation in HF. Venous return: High – normal – low (adapted from Mohrman, DE and Heller, LJ *Cardiovascular Physiology*, 4th ed. McGraw-Hill Comp., 1997, chapter 9, p. 147).

Under most physiological conditions, changes occur simultaneously in these relationships, although one effect will be dominant [37], for example:

- If CO rises with a fall in right atrial pressure (central venous pressure), the dominant effect is improvement in cardiac function (increase in contractility and/or reduction in afterload);
- If CO rises with an increase in RAP the dominant effect is an increase in volume, and a decrease in venous compliance or venous capacity, resulting in a higher venous flow for any pressure in the right atrium.

Remember that a decrease in venous resistance will enhance venous return [104] and that CVP and CO are determined by the interaction of the two functions, cardiac function and the venous return [38, 105, 106].

Hence, CVP can be **low** in a person with low blood volume and normal cardiac function, but it can also be low in cases of normal volume and good cardiac function [37].

CVP can be **high** in cases of normal filling with impaired cardiac function, but also in cases of normal function but with fluid overload [37].

While in the arterial system the pressure depends on, and is determined by, the **flow** and the arterial **resistance** (MAP = SV × SVR) [1], the venous blood flow is determined by considering **volume** and venous **capacitance** [107]:

$$\text{Total venous pressure (CVP) = volume × (fluid/venous) capacitance}$$

It is the **venous capacitance which dominates the venous behaviour** and the central venous pressure is determined, essentially, by the venous capacity [108, 109]. It is not the venous return (as a flow), but the **volume** that predominantly controls basic RAP/CVP [107].

During exercise, sympathetic activity stimulated by the reduced activity from arterial and atrial receptors will increase venous tone and decrease venous capacitance [110]. This will increase the venous return to the heart [111] and, in case of a recruitable preload reserve (this depends on CF [10, 11, 13, 82, 100, 103]), SV will increase [42, 43]. The immediate effect of a decrease in venous capacitance is an increase in all pressures [107], including transmural RVEDP and thus RV filling, enabling the RV to increase its systolic performance [42, 43].

**Fluid infusion** leads to **an increase in venous capacitance**, lowering the central venous pressure [109, 112, 113]. A high CVP always has consequences and will limit the venous return [49].

In patients with septic shock, Stephan [114] found that, despite vasodilatation of both the arterial and venous systems [115, 116], volume loading increased the venous tone and thus the CVP significantly and to high values (> 10 mm Hg). This is due to a marked reduction in the compliance of the venous system secondary to stiffening of the vein walls by several sepsis-induced mechanisms [114].

CVP is normally **0 mm Hg** at rest and might increase to **2–4 mm Hg** during exercise [117]. The **CVP is only elevated in disease states** [118, 119], a CVP > 10 mm Hg reflects an elevated RV-afterload [118].

In critically ill humans [4, 76, 102, 120, 121] as well as in healthy persons [83] we know that **no correlation at all exists between CVP and preload** or change in CVP and change in preload. The lack of a relationship is due to the fact that, in humans, the compliance of the atria and, in particular, of the ventricles is highly variable [83]. Furthermore, preload is not the same as fluid responsiveness [122, 123], and CVP and its change poorly (do not [124]) predict fluid responsiveness [10, 82, 125–128].

Thus, in daily practice the absolute value of the CVP and even dynamic changes in its value are very difficult to interpret and cannot be used as a valid indicator of fluid management at all [119].

In general, a CVP ≥ 10–12 mm Hg has to be considered high, and most patients within this range will not respond to volume administration [49]. Bafaqueeh [129] found that 40% of patients with a CVP < 6 mm Hg did not respond to further fluid administration.

Pericardial constraint accounts for 96% of the RAP, if CVP > 10 mm Hg [71]: A CVP ≥ 5 mm Hg [130], and particularly when exceeding 9–10 mm Hg, will exert substantial constraint on (left) ventricular filling [71, 131].

Thus, an **elevated CVP > 9–10 mm Hg** is **always** pathological [118, 119], signalling that fluid administration is unlikely to be successful [129] , and that **diastolic ventricular interaction (DVI)** [71, 131] may be present or will occur if the CVP increases further (see part 8 of this chapter).


## 1.4     Haemodynamic monitoring


## a)      Assessment and monitoring of fluid status

Haemodynamic monitoring is a cornerstone in the management of critically ill patients [119]. It helps identify pathological states [15, 132] and complications of circulatory failure [15, 119] and aids restoration of normal haemodynamic parameters to prevent tissue and organ injury, to restore organ failure/dysfunction and hence to reduce mortality [119].

When faced with a compromised circulation, volume expansion is very frequently the **first therapeutic measure** used to improve haemodynamic status [133]. Unfortunately, only 40–70% of all patients with acute circulatory failure respond to fluid administration (SV/CO ↑) [82], which means that 30–60% of patients are not fluid responsive and volume administration may be harmful [119, 134–136]. Both, acute and chronic right heart failure [52, 54] as well as acute left heart failure [26, 27] may deteriorate with volume loading.

Therefore a rational approach to fluid administration is needed, where the therapeutic decision is based on correctly assessed **effective intravascular volume** (preload) and the probable **response to increased volume** [119, 137]. However, the clinical tools available to evaluate the patient's fluid status and specifically the **intravascular/intraventricular filling (preload)**, such as jugular venous distension, crackles on auscultation, peripheral oedema, etc., are of minimal value and very poor indicators of the volume status, particularly in the critically ill patient with (cardiogenic) shock: They cannot be validated as a useful tool or basis for treatment decisions [138–146]. The only relevant clinical sign which, although still non-specific, may indicate a possible volume deficit is the **heart rate**. Volume deficits are usually compensated by an increase in heart rate (> 90 bpm) to maintain CO in case of low SV [101, 147, 148].

In acute heart failure patients a two-minute bedside assessment [96, 149, 150] is extremely helpful to allocate the patient to one specific haemodynamic profile (**wet or dry** *and* **cold or warm**) with corresponding treatment regimes [96, 150–152] (see detailed information in Chapter 2). This evaluation, however, does not provide any usable information about the patient's **actual intravascular fluid status** (to classify the patient as normo-, hypo-, or hypervolaemic) or whether a cold, and thus hypoperfused, patient will respond and benefit from fluids or not [33].

Hence, in addition to this useful bedside assessment, a proper assessment of the patient's intravascular volume status must be carried out to clarify whether a benefit (positive fluid responsiveness) can be expected from volume expansion **before** fluids are given. Blind administration of intravenous fluid may be harmful through an increase in LVEDP [134], as the elevation of the LVEDP predominantly causes the patient's symptoms to worsen [97] and, with increasing LVEDP, the patient's prognosis [17, 96, 97].

In case of central hypovolaemia, volume administration will induce a significant increase in SV (flow) **as long as a preload reserve can be recruited** [134, 135, 153, 154]. Thus, it is important to predict in a haemodynamically unstable patient whether this patient will increase his/her systemic blood flow (SV) in response to volume expansion or not [135].

Kumar [9] showed that, in healthy individuals, volume loading increases the systolic BP/ LVESV ratio and the LV-SW by:

- an increase in LV-SV due to a reduction in LVESV while the LVEDV remains unchanged and
- an increase in contractility.

The contribution of the Frank–Starling mechanism is only mild to moderate; the contractility is the main component [9]. Kumar examined healthy volunteers and confirmed the findings of animal studies conducted in the 1960–70s [155–157]. Flow represented by SV is the original, central, and decisive parameter to be assessed when defining fluid responsiveness [82, 83, 123, 135, 153, 158].

**Fluid loading must increase LV-SV if the heart is preload responsive** [82, 135, 153].

In heart failure, although the LVEDV may be in the normal range, fluid administration can fail

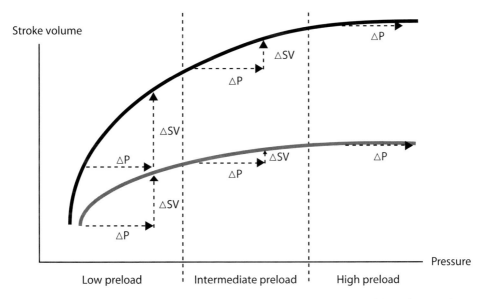

**Figure 1.4** Δp: change in filling pressure; ΔSV: change in SV; upper curve: normal heart function, lower curve: impaired heart function (modified from Michard, F [10]).

to increase the SV due to a significant reduction in contractility [10, 82, 100, 101]. Furthermore, we know that the Frank–Starling mechanism is impaired in heart failure [56, 99] and hence volume expansion may well be harmful and worsen the haemodynamic situation [119, 134–136].

Braunwald [100], and recently Michard [10, 82] have established proof that **the increase in SV due to increased LVEDV depends on the contractility and pre-infusion preload** (initial end-diastolic fibre length in respect to the Frank–Starling mechanism), **particularly in the case of compromised cardiac function** [10, 82, 100].

In those patients with intermediate pre-infusion preload (normovolemia), the effect of volume loading depends exclusively on the contractility and, in the case of a compromised heart function (lower curve) in 'intermediate preloaded' patients, the effect of volume loading in order to increase SV, and thus CO and/or BP, is minimal and clinically not relevant [10].

Nevertheless, even in cases of cardiogenic or other types of shock, fluid administration may **initially** be helpful. Up to 70% of all patients in shock show a positive response (increase of blood pressure, increasing the perfusion of vital organs) when fluids are administered [159]. In non-responders we most often find that RV-dysfunction/failure with sepsis is the main underlying reason [159].

The physiological and pathophysiological facts described above demonstrate and emphasise that preload and fluid responsiveness are not the same, and this has been stressed in many published studies [119, 122, 123, 134, 160]. Therefore, as prerequisites to a **positive response** to fluid administration, there must exist both a recruitable contractile reserve (**myocardial reserve**) and an absolute or relatively hypovolaemic **central vascular and cardiac system** to provide a filling reserve.

An increase in SV by ≥ 15% due to volume administration is the most accepted benchmark confirming a positive fluid response [125, 126, 161–163], although others define a positive response if SV increases secondary to volume expansion by ≥ 10% [154, 164–167].

## b)        Prediction of fluid responsiveness

### i)        Pressure measurements
**Cardiac filling pressures** such as CVP and LVEDP/PCWP have **failed** to predict either preload or fluid responsiveness. The relationship (if there is any) between the intravascular/intraventricular volume and the CVP/PCWP is, as already mentioned, very poor in both ill patients [4, 76, 120, 121, 168, 169] and healthy volunteers [83]. Even in sedated and mechanically ventilated patients, CVP and PCWP have been shown to be unreliable parameters to reflect the preload or to predict fluid responsiveness [10, 82, 83, 125, 127, 128, 170]. Osman [124] states that, "fluid responsiveness is documented to be unrelated to CVP/RAP and PCWP/LVEDP, respectively".

### ii)        Volumetric measurements
**Volumetric measurements** (RVEDV, ITBV or GEDV) and **ventricular areas** (LVEDA or LVEDD) have been shown to **be useful in assessing the preload** and seem to be better than cardiac filling pressures in guiding volume therapy [82, 83, 171, 172] but, unfortunately, they are still not great at predicting **fluid responsiveness** [125, 126, 173, 174].

In particular, it was hoped that GEDV(I), reflecting central blood volume [175, 176], and the direct measurement of the RVEDV would overcome the mentioned difficulties. However, the indirectly measured volumetric parameter GEDV **failed** to provide additional prediction in terms of the patient's response to volume expansion [9, 171, 172, 177]. The direct measurement of the absolute value of the RVEDV allows a definitive assessment of volume status, however unfortunately whilst SV increased with volume loading there was no change in the measured RVEDV [9].

Furthermore, Reuter found only a poor correlation between SV and LVEDA (from echocardiography) [165], and Slama showed that changes in LVEDD are also dependent on LV stiffness [178]. Several other authors followed by confirming the poor correlation between LVEDD and SV/CO [126, 162, 168].

Thus, filling pressures such as CVP/RAP, PCWP, or areas/geometric dimensions of the LV, such as LVEDA or LVEDD, are unable to predict fluid responsiveness [82, 119], nor can direct [9] or indirect measurements of end-diastolic volumes [overview by 82] predict the patient's response to volume expansion [171, 172, 177].

**Preload is simply not the same as preload responsiveness [119, 123, 134, 160, 179].**

Osman concludes that, in the assessment of preload responsiveness, parameters other than pressures and ventricular volumes need to be measured [124].

### iii)      Dynamic parameters
In contrast to the static parameters discussed above for assessing the filling pressures, filling volumes, and left ventricular areas, we have the **dynamic parameters,** which comprise stroke volume variation (SV-V), pulse pressure variation (PP-V), systolic blood pressure variation (SP-V) and aortic blood flow changes, which provide substantial information and are valuable tools in predicting fluid responsiveness [125, 126, 161, 162, 172, 180, 181].

The dynamic parameters reflect changes in LV-SV due to heart-lung interactions induced by mechanical ventilation [125, 126, 147, 177, 182–185] and several studies have documented that variations in LV-SV associated with mechanical ventilation are highly predictive of preload responsiveness [125, 161, 162, 165, 178, 186].

The alterations in cardiac preload, and hence variations in LV-SV associated with respiration, are referred as to SV-V and are defined by the maximum to minimum SV values during a period of three breaths, or over a time interval of 20 to 30 seconds [162, 167, 178]. SV-V is validated in several studies for deeply sedated, mechanically ventilated patients with a tidal volume of 6 ml/kg without any spontaneous breathing effort. A SV-V ≥ 10% predicts an increase in CO of ≥ 15% for a 500 ml fluid bolus [166, 167, 178].

Positive pressure ventilation with its cyclic increases in intrathoracic pressure and lung volume [187, 188] induces intermittent variations in cardiac preload (heart-lung interaction) [165, 189–191]. This is predominantly due to a reduction in venous return secondary to the increase in RA pressure during mechanical inspiration [189, 192–194]; hence, the RV filling is reduced (↓ RVEDV) [189, 195–197]. In accordance with the Frank–Starling mechanism this produces a reduction in RV-SV [42, 43, 125]. An additional effect that is at least partly responsible for the reduction in RV-SV is exerted by the increase in RV-outflow impedance [198, 199] and thus a rise in RV-afterload with consecutive impaired RV ejection secondary to positive pressure ventilation [191, 200–202].

However, this inspiratory reduction in RV-SV affects the LV-filling after a few heart beats, producing a ↓ LVEDV [190, 203, 204]. Consequently, the LV-SV is reduced [190, 191, 203, 204] and this takes effect during expiration. Thus, ventilation-dependent variations in RV-filling will induce cyclic variations in LV-filling with a concomitant reduction in LV-SV, and thus arterial blood pressure, if both RV and LV are fluid responsive [125, 119, 191, 203].

Conversely, during inspiration the opposite occurs; increased LV-filling will result in a higher LVEDV and hence higher LV-SV and arterial pressure [119, 191, 203].

The influence of positive pressure ventilation on the cyclic haemodynamic changes is greater when central blood volume is low rather than when it is normal or high [82, 139, 162, 205].

The dynamic parameters will lose their validity if tidal volumes vary from breath to breath, as with (assisted) spontaneous breathing [135, 164, 206] or in case of marked arrhythmias inducing variations in LV-SV [139]. Exaggerated values of SV-V were found with large tidal volumes, reduced chest wall compliance and air trapping [165]. Furthermore, a moderately elevated intra-abdominal pressure (up to 20 cm $H_2O$) affects cyclic circulatory changes by inducing a progressive increase in intrathoracic pressure enhancing the pleural pressure swings and thus may feign fluid responsiveness [207]; if the intra-abdominal pressure is higher than 20 cm $H_2O$, less influence is seen [207].

Nevertheless, the dynamic parameters have shown themselves to be far better than the static parameters in predicting fluid responsiveness and are currently the approach of choice in sedated and ventilated patients [119, 139, 161, 162, 164, 165].

The **dynamic swing** in LV-**SV** is the current gold standard [153, 161] in predicting response to fluid administration – but SV-V, although affected by preload, predominantly also seems to reflect the **myocardial response** to volume loading [165]. This is consistent with our knowledge that SV predominantly depends on LV-function (mainly the contractility [10, 82, 100, 101] and, in heart failure, on afterload as well [11–13, 51, 103]) rather than on pre-infusion preload [10, 82, 100]. Kumar [9] showed that, in healthy volunteers, the increase in SV due to volume loading is predominantly a result of an increase in contractility rather than an increase in filling volume, and thus a larger fibre stretch as described by Frank and Starling.

Besides the assessment of SV-V during positive pressure mechanical ventilation [206], surrogates of SV such as aortic flow [162, 166], systolic BP (SP-V) [203, 208], and pulse pressure (PP-V) [125, 153] have turned out to be reliable and valuable indices by which to check central blood volume and the response to fluid administration.

*Descending aortic blood flow as a direct correlate of SV/CO*
Descending aortic blood flow represents the majority of CO [209, 210] and is accepted as a clinically realistic estimate of SV and or CO [211–213]. Aortic Doppler flow velocity measurements can determine the SV, calculated with the help of the product of the velocity-time interval in the ascending (estimated by echocardiography [160]) or descending aorta (oesophageal Doppler measurement) [212, 214–216] and a measured [160] or estimated aortic diameter using the nomogram by Boulnois [217]. These flow velocity measurements have been reported to predict fluid responsiveness accurately [162, 178, 212, 216].

*Systolic pressure variation (SP-V)*
Systolic pressure variation (SP-V) is probably the easiest way to assess fluid responsiveness and is defined as an 'increase or decrease in systolic arterial pressure with each mechanical breath relative to the systolic pressure during the short apnoea phase' [208, 218]. Numerous studies

have shown its value as a sensitive parameter in predicting preload responsiveness in patients who are mechanically ventilated without any spontaneous breathing [126, 162, 165, 177, 180, 218–221]. The sensitivity of this method is not as high as that of PP-V because it does not quantify the varying diastolic arterial pressure components [125].

*Pulse pressure variation (PP-V)*
Pulse pressure variation (PP-V) may be the most robust and sensitive indirect indicator of volume status [82, 125]. The variation of the aortic pulse pressure (aortic pulse pressure ~ LV-SV [222, 223]) is established as an evidence-based index with which to assess and predict the response to fluid administration in mechanically ventilated patients [82]. A cyclic variation of the aortic pulse pressure due to varying LV-SV during a respiratory cycle of more than 13% ($r^2$ = 0.85, p < 0.001) [82] implies a very high likelihood (85%) that the patient will benefit from fluid administration with a significant increase in SV and thus in blood pressure (positive predictive value of 94%, negative predictive value of 96%) [82, 204, 224].

Calculation of PP-V during one respiratory cycle:
$Pp_{max}$: maximal systolic pressure – maximal diastolic pressure,
$Pp_{min}$: minimal systolic pressure – minimal diastolic pressure.
$$\textbf{PPV (\%)} = [(\textbf{Pp}_{max} - \textbf{Pp}_{min}) \ / \ (\textbf{Pp}_{max} + \textbf{Pp}_{min})/2] \times \textbf{100}.$$

*Passive leg raising (PLR), an autotransfusion of fluids*
Several studies recently published have given encouraging evidence that prediction of fluid response is feasible in spontaneously breathing as well as ventilated patients [134, 160].

Raising the legs to approximately 30 or 45 degrees is called passive leg raising (PLR) and will increase the aortic flow **in case of a recruitable preload reserve** 15 to 60 seconds after the legs have been raised [135, 153, 158, 160] and this will persist for 30 to 90 seconds [225] (Pinsky [119] up to three minutes).

Clinical studies have proven that the volume of blood transferred to the heart by PLR is sufficient to increase the left ventricular filling volume [135, 153, 226–229]. While the predictive value of the transient changes in SV is only fair if SV or its surrogates, SP-V and PP-V, are estimated from a **peripheral pulse** pressure curve [133, 135] – due to the influence of the arterial compliance and the vasomotor tone [153, 223] – high sensitivities were achieved when measuring **variations in SV centrally**, i.e. by oesophageal Doppler [135], echocardiography [160] or by femoral artery access, which is considered to be central [230, 231]: Monnet [135] found a sensitivity of 97% and a specificity of 94% to achieve an increase of ≥ 15% in aortic blood flow in response to volume administration if, during PLR, the aortic blood flow increased by ≥ 10%. Lamia [160] showed a similar specificity (100%) but with a slightly worse (but still good) sensitivity of 77%.

Thus, an increase in aortic blood flow (SV/CO) by ≥ 10% [135, 153, 154] or 12.5% [160] during PLR is reliably predictive of central hypovolaemia and a positive response to volume expansion [153, 134, 135, 154, 160] in either mechanically ventilated patients or those breathing spontaneously. In the **absence of central hypovolaemia** and/or in the presence of an **unresponsive RV and/or LV** (compromised function, mainly impaired contractility) SV/CO will not increase by the PLR manoeuvre [135, 153, 154].

As no external fluids are administered, the hazards of unnecessary volume loading can be avoided [49, 95, 172, 232–238] and hence the measurement of **central blood flow** (aortic blood flow normally represented by SV or CO) in response to **PLR** is more robust and probably **superior** to PP-V when **evaluating the patients' fluid response**, even in spontaneously breathing patients [123, 134, 135, 160]. Furthermore, this approach is more independent of varying tidal volumes and arrhythmias than a peripheral one [134, 135, 160]. The central measurement of blood flow avoids the relevant influences of arterial compliance and vasomotor tone [223] and the complex changes in pulse wave propagation and reflection along the arterial vessel system [239], both of which may change during PLR with a concomitant change in SV.

### iv)      Fluid challenge

A fluid challenge is still advocated as a tool to evaluate the need for further fluid administration if strictly monitored and the response observed closely [137, 240], but the dynamic parameters described above are clearly superior and blind volume administration should be avoided if at all possible [134].

A fluid challenge does not mean fluid resuscitation; it merely identifies those patients who are likely to show a beneficial response to (further) fluid administration [241].

To minimise the amount of fluid needed to assess responsiveness, the fluid should be given quickly [49] and some authors require an increase in CVP of at least 2 mm Hg [242, 243] to confirm that a sufficient amount of fluid has been given. Rapid bolus administration of 250 ml in 5–7 min or 500 ml in 10 min [49] of fluid or PLR is expected to show an appropriate haemodynamic response if beneficial for the patient [118, 242]. If a recruitable preload reserve is available, the SV must increase [242].

Although no definition as to what comprises an adequate fluid challenge is generally agreed upon, most studies do agree that a positive response is indicated by improving circulatory status as suggested by ↑ BP, heart rate unchanged or ↓, with accompanying SV ↑, and an improved effective blood flow documented by $ScvO_2/SvO_2$ ↑, and lactate ↓ [118].

It is always worth remembering that a fluid challenge should only be performed if an indication is obvious, i.e. within the context of hypoperfusion [244] and that there is only a very poor correlation between change in BP and CO [49]. If no positive effect is achieved, fluid administration is useless, potentially harmful, and must be stopped immediately [49, 95, 172, 232–238].

Despite uncertainty, even in life-threatening situations such as cardiogenic shock, the administration of moderate amounts of fluid (about 3 ml/kg, hence ~ 250–300 ml) as a fluid challenge under close monitoring is appropriate and may stabilise the acute situation **temporarily** [245]. Appropriate and immediate fluid resuscitation in critically ill patients, if adequate, will improve outcome [246]. McConachie [247] states that a fluid challenge is appropriate in virtually all critically ill patients in shock situations with blood pressure 'too' low and/or hypoperfusion due to low cardiac output, unless obviously suffering from gross congestive cardiac failure.

On the other hand, it must be emphasised that, although a patient responds to volume administration, this does not automatically mean that the patient requires volume, as healthy subjects will respond as well [49, 241].

Vincent and Weil have recently proposed the following algorithm as being the proper approach to performing a fluid challenge [137]. In hypotensive patients with circulatory compromise administer 250–500 ml colloidal fluid (~ 3–5 ml/kg) over 15–20 min in order to stabilise the patient haemodynamically (at least temporarily), to improve organ and tissue perfusion, and to 'test the system' as to whether or not they are likely to respond positively to further fluid administration.

Criteria suggestive of effective volume loading [10, 37, 125, 137, 232, 244]:
- **increase in SV by ≥ 10% and/or increase in systolic blood pressure by ≥ 10%,**
- heart rate unchanged or reduced,
- **CVP increase ≤ 2–5 mm Hg** (if > 5, no further administration, be cautious already if increase > 2),
- no clinical signs of fluid overload,
- additional parameters, if monitored:
  - PCWP increase ≤ 3–7 mm Hg; stop fluids if increase > 7 mm Hg,
  - EVLWI prior and post fluids ≤ 7–10 ml/kg,
  - ↓ lactate, positive result by OPS (see below),
  - increase in urinary output.

**Stop** fluid challenge during or after infusion if [10, 37, 125, 137, 232, 244]:
- **SV/blood pressure does not increase appropriately** (< 10%) [101, 147, 148];
- **Hypoperfusion does not improve** (clinically, no ↑ UO, no ↓ lactate / no ↑ SaO$_2$, no change in capnography / OPS evidence of improved tissue perfusion);
- **CVP increase > 5 mm Hg** due to volume administration, be cautious if increase > 2: ↑ risk for DVI;
- **High risk of DVI** if CVP > 9–10 mm Hg [131, 118, 119, 248] and particularly if SV/BP falls during volume administration.
- Additional parameters, if monitored:
  - EVLWI > 10 ml/kg [214, 249–251],
  - PCWP-increase > 7 mm Hg.

An International Consensus Conference [243] from 2006 suggested 'a rise in CVP of at least 2 mm Hg either by 250 ml fluid administration within 10–15 min, or leg raising' as a sign of sufficient fluid administration – defining a positive response if cardiac function and tissue perfusion improve. However, bear in mind that this recommendation is non-specific and expert opinion only.

As we know, CVP does not reflect preload or changes in preload, either in healthy or critically ill patients [76, 83, 120, 121, 168, 169]. Thus, CVP cannot be used as a predictor of RV-filling and cannot be used to assess the effect of volume loading. A change in the magnitude of the CVP of at least 2 mm Hg is the minimum necessary for detection with confidence on most currently used monitors [49] and therefore seems to be an arbitrary figure. Remember, in patients with good cardiac function, the CVP may even fall despite the fluid challenge being successful [83] and, if using the PLR method, central monitoring is essential and peripheral monitoring is not adequate [133].

**v)     PiCCO-monitoring (Pulse-induced continuous cardiac output)**
PiCCO is a method of haemodynamic monitoring which combines transpulmonary thermodilution and continuous arterial pulse contour analysis (see overview by Pfeiffer [252]).

This method allows the measurement of volumes [40, 170, 253] such as intra-thoracic blood volume (ITBV) representing the intra-vascular volume status, the global end-diastolic volume GEDV (of all four chambers) and, of most importance, the extra-vascular lung water (EVLW) [233, 249, 254].

These **volumetric** measurements are performed semi-invasively and are superior to the common pressure measurements, CVP and PCWP, when assessing the patient's intravascular volume status and the cardiac preload [93, 94, 120, 255]. Unfortunately, these parameters (ITBV and GEDV) do not allow any prediction of the response of the circulatory system to fluid administration [82, 171, 172] (see above). However, the PiCCO-method fulfils all the requirements to evaluate response from PLR [135, 160, 256].

EVLW is an extremely informative parameter, proven as being an accurate measurement of the real amount of fluid in the lung tissue [233, 250, 254], the EVLW value provides substantial information about patient prognosis [233–235, 249]. Currently, it is the only method able to diagnose 'developing' pulmonary oedema earlier than all other available methods, including clinical examination, chest X-ray and pressure measurement via PA-catheter (PCWP) [120, 234, 257–260]. Furthermore, it is able to guide investigation of the pathologically high lung water: cardiac or extra-cardiac causes [238, 254, 261, 262].

Two-thirds of all HF patients with a mean PCWP of < 18 mm Hg (18 mm Hg is the generally accepted upper limit in case of a failing heart, probably providing the maximum preload recruitable SV) show a significantly increased EVLW/EVLWI [263], although it is not detectable by auscultation or on X-ray [145, 264]. On the other hand, the PCWP is measured to be

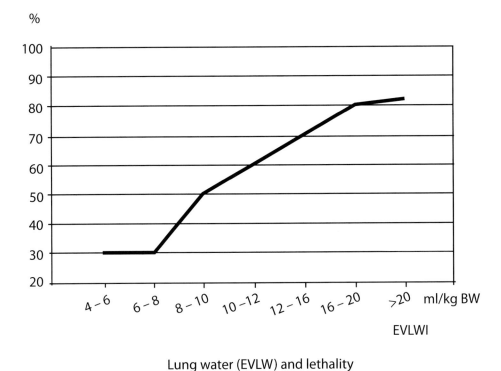

Lung water (EVLW) and lethality

**Figure 1.5** This diagram shows the mortality rate depending on the amount of extravascular lung water. The graph is of special value because it is validated by post mortem analysis of lung water, confirming the accuracy of the clinical measurement (adapted from Sturm et al. [233]).

normal ($\leq 12$ mm Hg) in some cases of cardiogenic shock, particularly in previously healthy patients with acute myocardial infarction, but the EVLW is already elevated and thus pulmonary oedema is present [33, 265–267]. An increased EVLW/EVLWI signals increased mortality [233–235, 268] and in the case of an elevated EVLW, any fluid reduction will lead to an increase in CO [269].

EVLW is valuable in indicating fluid overload [250, 259, 260] and its value (normal range EVLWI 3–7 ml/kg) should influence your therapeutic decision. If the EVLWI exceeds 10 ml/kg, the mortality increases exponentially and further fluid administration is not advisable [233, 236, 268, 251].

The permeability index PVPI (PVPI = EVLW/pulmonary blood volume (PBV) with PBV = ITBV – GEDV) reflects, if elevated (> 3), an increased capillary permeability (capillary leakage resulting in non-cardiogenic oedema) [238, 254, 261, 262], while an index < 3 in combination of elevated EVLW/I is suggestive for a cardiogenic oedema.

**vi)  Echocardiography**

Echocardiography is essential to help diagnose the underlying pathology in circulatory failure and/or cardiac dysfunction [270, 271]. Heidenreich [272] successfully improved diagnostic accuracy by identifying a further 28% of the underlying aetiologies in unexplained hypotension when examining patients by transoesophageal echocardiography (TOE) in addition to the other obtained hemodynamic parameters. Thus, he showed that TOE adds significant information to invasively acquired haemodynamic data. Echocardiography has the ability to rapidly diagnose and aid decisive therapeutic decisions in cases of cardiac tamponade [273] and aortic dissection [274], confirming the clinically suggested diagnosis of endocarditis [275], to reveal evidence of haemodynamically significant pulmonary embolism [276], and is, of course, extremely helpful in assessing the heart's performance [277].

The assessment and evaluation of SV/CO, probably the main determinant of sufficient organ perfusion, is relatively easy to obtain by flow measurement in the descending aorta [214]. Laupland [215 ] gave proof that this is easy, quick to learn, and simply done in daily practice. However, this method does have some limitations. It is assumed that about 70% of the total CO will reach the descending aorta [217] and, furthermore, instead of measuring the diameter of the LVOT needed for the calculation of CO, a nomogram by Boulnois [217] is used. Thus, this method provides a rough estimate of the CO and the correlations with invasive measurements are weak when compared with PA-catheterisation or PiCCO [268, 278, 279]. If estimating the CO with PA catheterisation, as recommended by the ESC and AHA, advanced skills and training are necessary [280, 281].

There have been 11 large studies evaluating the use of echocardiography as a continuous monitoring method in critically ill patients, most of them using the transoesophageal technique. No final conclusion can be made as to whether or not echocardiography should be recommended as equal to the established methods in continuous haemodynamic monitoring. Echocardiography is time consuming, requires advanced physician training in acquisition and interpretation, and it is not realistic to establish this technology on a 24 hour basis worldwide [282–284]. The usefulness of echocardiography lies in its diagnostic capacity and there is a consensus that an echocardiogram is absolutely essential in the initial assessment of all patients suffering from (cardiogenic) shock and should be performed as early as possible [270, 271, 285, 286]. Echocardiography (especially TOE) frequently depicts abnormalities overlooked by catheter-based invasive assessment tools such as LVOT obstruction, diastolic ventricular interaction,

RV-dysfunction/failure, LV diastolic dysfunction, valve disease, cardiac compression, etc. [272, 287]. Furthermore, it has a great impact on therapeutic considerations, with 60% [288] of planned treatments altered following echocardiography [288–292].

Echocardiography can be a life saving tool; in cardiac failure patients, echocardiography is far easier and faster than PA-catheterisation and provides key haemodynamic information [293].

## c)      Arterial blood pressure

### i)      BP and autoregulation

Adequate organ perfusion is essential to avoid the development of shock [294]. Although the mean arterial pressure (MAP) is the best estimate of organ perfusion pressure [118], there is no known threshold pressure defining adequate perfusion pressure amongst different organs, between patients, or in a patient over time [295]. The autoregulation of most organs maintains a constant organ-specific blood flow over a broad range of varying BPs and changes in metabolic rates, but hypotension is always pathological [118, 119].

Most authors define hypotension as systolic BP < 90 mm Hg [296, 297], MAP ≤ 65 [295, 298] to 70 mm Hg [299–301], although in known hypertensive patients this may be altered to a MAP ≤ 85 mm Hg and, in known hypotensive patients, ≤ 50–60 mm Hg. In patients with IHD a MAP of ≤ 75–80 mm Hg [295, 302–304] is commonly used.

Hypotension impairs autoregulated blood flow distribution [305, 306], and the MAP needed to maintain autoregulation varies from organ to organ and depends on clinical conditions (i.e. known arteriosclerotic disease or not).

*Kidneys*
A constant renal blood flow is maintained by autoregulation, which acts in a range of MAPs between 80–180 mm Hg [307–310]. Iglesias [311] demands a MAP > 70 mm Hg in order to prevent acute renal failure, or if acute kidney injury has already developed, in order to re-establish adequate renal perfusion. Esson [312] stresses that adequate renal perfusion pressure is a cornerstone of care in acute renal failure.

*Brain*
Autoregulation works within MAPs of 60–160 mm Hg [313]; the recommendations for an adequate cerebral perfusion pressure in critical illness vary from at least 60 mm Hg [314, 315] to ≥ 70 mm Hg [313, 316].

**Cerebral perfusion pressure = MAP – (Intra-cerebral pressure + CVP)**

(In case of brain injury even higher pressures may be desirable).

*Heart*
A coronary perfusion pressure (CPP) of > 50 mm Hg is essential for the basic supply of the myocardium [317, 318].

**CPP = diastolic blood pressure – LVEDP [319]**

Coronary autoregulation functions from (50 [302]) 60 mm Hg up to 140 mm Hg [302, 303]. This means that in the case of an elevated LVEDP (> 15 mm Hg), a **minimal diastolic pressure** of > 65 mm Hg is essential. In coronary artery disease, even higher pressures are required in order to prevent further deterioration due to progressive ischaemia [295, 302–304].

*Septic Shock*
In septic shock, a MAP between ≥ 65 mm Hg [298, 304, 320, 321] and 75 mm Hg (in patients with known occlusive arterial disease, peripheral arteriosclerosis or long standing hypertension) [304] is recommended. A study by LeDoux showed that a MAP between 65 mm Hg and 85 mm Hg was not associated with significant differences in organ perfusion [295].

This was confirmed by Bourgoin [298] who showed that an increase in MAP from 65 mm Hg to 85 mm Hg with an infusion of noradrenaline did not improve **renal function**. The key point is that, as long as autoregulation is not substantially disturbed, a MAP of ≥ 65 mm Hg is sufficient. But in case of a breakdown of autoregulation, however, higher MAPs are necessary to re-install it [298].

However, even a BP generally considered normal does not necessarily reflect haemodynamic stability and adequate organ perfusion [322]. Blood pressure is an inadequate indicator of incipient shock in a patient [323]. It is therefore essential to make an assessment of tissue perfusion.

**ii)      Assessment of tissue perfusion**
Organ perfusion essentially depends on blood flow and thus cardiac function [214]. Circulatory shock is known to cause tissue hypoperfusion [119] and inadequate tissue perfusion is associated with elevated morbidity and mortality [246, 324–329].

Compared to the difficult task of evaluating the vascular fluid status and the patient's likely response to volume expansion, tissue hypoperfusion can be assessed fairly well by clinical examination [285, 297, 330]. Clinical signs suggestive of tissue hypoperfusion are [133, 134, 160]:
- tachycardia,
- hypotension (sBP < 90 mm Hg, MAP < 70 (60) mm Hg, or BP-drop > 40 mm Hg),
- oligo-/anuria,
- clinical or biological signs of extracellular fluid depletion (ketoacidosis, vomiting, diarrhoea),
- delayed capillary refill,
-  mottled skin,
-  altered level of consciousness.

Menon [285] strongly recommends **a diagnosis** of cardiogenic shock (CS) in all patients exhibiting *signs of inadequate tissue perfusion* in the setting of severe cardiac dysfunction **irrespective of the BP**.

$SvO_2$ (mixed venous oxygen saturation) reflects the balance between oxygen delivery and oxygen consumption [331, 332]. Pinsky [119] and Reinhart [333] state that a decrease in $SvO_2$ to < 70% represents increased oxygen extraction by the tissues [119, 333] suggestive of hypoperfusion [334]. A persistent $SvO_2$ < 30% is associated with severe tissue ischaemia [335].

Plasma lactate levels, although non-specific, are still a reasonable surrogate for inadequate tissue perfusion [336–338]. A reduction of an initially elevated value signals improvement of perfusion [339].

Thus, ↑ plasma lactate levels and ↓ $SvO_2$ [340, 341] coupled with a suggestive clinical examination may help support the **earlier** diagnosis of tissue hypoxia.

Ander [342] found that monitoring of $ScvO_2$ and lactate in patients with severe heart failure (patients with known cardiomyopathy being admitted with acute decompensation) is superior to assessment and monitoring clinical vital signs for the recognition of occult cardiogenic shock. If both parameters are abnormal (lactate > 2 mmol/l, $ScvO_2$ < 60%), occult/pre-cardiogenic shock requiring a special therapeutic approach could be clearly identified, whilst this was not possible from the vital signs [342].

Newer developments such as *sublingual capnography* [343, 344], *orthogonal polarization spectral spectroscopy (OPS)* [345, 346] and *near-infrared spectroscopy (NIRS)* attempt to measure local tissue blood flow and oxygen utilisation [347, 348] and evaluate any improvement due to therapeutic intervention.

Due to the fact that the use of 'the conventional global haemodynamic and oxygenation approach' may fail to provide adequate information on tissue perfusion, non-invasive monitoring of peripheral perfusion could become complementary in acting to warn of imminent global tissue hypoxia [349].

It must be remembered that the rationale for haemodynamic monitoring is to restore normal haemodynamic parameters in order to prevent organ injury and restore organ dysfunction [119]; however this may not be valid in all cases. Haemodynamic monitoring usually assesses the **global** circulatory status, **not** organ function or **microcirculation** [350–352], and does not address the mechanisms by which disease occurs [353, 354]. Therefore, we have to be careful in drawing therapeutic conclusions from the results of monitoring the macrocirculation; improvement of macrocirculation may compromise the microcirculation even further [355].

## 1.5    Afterload

### a)    Definition

The **force opposing fibre shortening during ventricular ejection is called afterload** [36, 356–358].

Myocardial wall stress during contraction **represents** 'true' **afterload**, because the wall stress reflects the combined effects of **central aortic and peripheral loading conditions** as well as the **intrinsic properties** within the heart itself [357, 359–361].

### b)    Estimation, measurements and interpretation

Braunwald [362] states that the (after) **load opposing LV ejection** in its simplest sense is reflected in the systolic blood pressure. However, the physiology is much more complex and systolic blood pressure has turned out to be a very poor reflection of afterload [363]. The tension that the ventricular wall sarcomeres must overcome during systole in order to shorten is related to [362, 364, 365]:

- characteristics of the arterial system [364–366],
- LV cavity size described by the law of LaPlace [365, 367] (see below),
- pumping performance of the LV. Systolic LV function and LV afterload are interrelated and the volume ejected is greater with a more vigorous LV contraction.

**LaPlace's law** mediates the relationship between end-systolic wall stress as a measure of 'true' myocardial afterload and the specific ventricular conditions during, and at, end-systole (diameter, LV pressure, and wall thickness) [365, 368–370]:

**Wall stress (tension) = LV (RV) pressure × LV (RV) diameter/2 × wall thickness [368]**

Dilatation will induce an increase in LV(RV) diameter and/or increasing LV(RV) pressure leads to a rise in wall stress and vice versa. An increase in wall thickness (in the case of hypertrophy) reduces the wall stress.

**LV dilatation → increasing wall stress/tension [368, 371]**

It must be emphasised that, due to LaPlace's law, LV wall stress reflects both vascular loading conditions and intrinsic heart muscle properties such as LV-geometry and intracavitary pressure [356, 359]. Determinants of the LV wall stress mediated by LaPlace's law are continuously changing during systole, producing varying measurements of LV wall stress depending on the phase of the cardiac cycle. Peak wall stress occurs within the first third of ejection, and wall stress then declines to its end-systolic value, which is less than 50% of the peak value. At the same time, the total systolic wall stress (estimated by the stress time integral) predicts myocardial oxygen consumption [372, 373].

All measures show a significant difference and the choice of index depends on the question being asked [373]
- total stress reflects myocardial oxygen consumption,
- peak stress correlates closely with the progress of hypertrophy,
- end-systolic wall stress represents most accurately the afterload.

The **very good correlation** between **end-systolic wall stress** and **myocardial fibre length at end-systole** [76] as well as between **end-systolic wall stress** and **end-systolic ventricular volume** (ESV) [374–377] underlines the fact that the *end-systolic wall stress is literally the (after)load* that limits the ejection [378, 379].

**Afterload ~ end-systolic wall stress and ~ end-systolic volume [368, 374–376].**

Furthermore, several authors have confirmed the excellent correlation in daily practice between end-systolic wall stress and LV afterload [357, 361, 375, 376, 380].

During systole the LV-chamber size will decrease while the ventricle contracts and thus the wall tension will fall. When the afterload increases, a greater pressure rise for any given reduction in chamber size is necessary and, therefore, wall tension during systole is higher. The pressure rise has to increase even more, of course, in a primarily dilated LV [20].

There are two echocardiographic methods described by Reichek [370] (M-mode assessment, meridional wall stress) and Greim [381] (2D-assessment, circumferential wall stress) which directly assess the end-systolic wall stress. Both are time consuming, require advanced skills, and Greim [381] expresses concerns about the ability of the M-mode method to recognise acute changes in afterload in patients during cardiothoracic surgery.

In daily practice the **systemic (peripheral) vascular resistance** (SVR) is the most common parameter used to describe the actual afterload, and often SVR is used synonymously with afterload.

SVR, however, only reflects the non-pulsatile component of the peripheral load under steady state conditions [382]. It does not comprise the impact of wave reflections, arterial impedance, or ventricular ejection gradients. Each of these phenomena augments LV-afterload independently of peripheral vascular resistance or arterial pressure [361]. Ageing, hypertension, and aortic stiffening contribute considerably to the pulsatile component of the afterload and thus this component becomes more prominent under those conditions [383, 384].

Lang [385] showed in his investigation that the measurement of SVR substantially underestimates the change in afterload when LV afterload alone was decreased, increased, or decreased, but with a simultaneous increase in contractility.

These findings are not surprising because, from the peripheral pressure-flow relationship, the **systemic peripheral resistance** is **not seen by the LV** [370].

Nevertheless, SVR accounts for 95% of the resistance to ejection (arterial resistance is the dominant component of impedance load [386]), and thus is justified as being the most commonly used parameter to clinically estimate afterload [363]. Furthermore, SVR may be very helpful in clarifying the diagnosis [15, 132, 363], particularly in hypotensive patients and in heart failure syndromes as shown by Cotter [15].

LV-afterload is well reflected by the **effective arterial elastance** $(E_a)$. The functional properties of the vascular system, the so-called **arterial load** (arterial input impedance [387, 388]) **faced** by the **ventricle during systole**, is **generally** accepted, as being **described by the effective arterial elastance** [389–391]. Being independent of actual cardiac output [392–394], $E_a$ reflects not only the peripheral and central resistance but the pulsatile component of the vessel system as well [395, 396]. Variations in the vascular diameter, in particular vasodilatation of the large arteries, are not reflected by the SVR, but are by $E_a$ [397].

$E_a$ is defined as left ventricular end-systolic pressure (LVESP) divided by stroke volume (SV) [389, 390];

$$E_a = LVESP/SV = sBP \times 0.9/SV,$$

where sBP (systolic arterial pressure) equals the end-systolic left ventricular pressure when multiplied by 0.9 [390]. Normal value, $E_a \approx 2.0$ mm Hg/ml [390, 398–400].

Kelly established proof that $E_a$ and its changes correlate very well with varying loading and inotropic conditions, reflecting relative effects of vasodilation on cardiac performance adequately and, so, predicting effects and benefits of therapy [401].

## c)  Afterload in acute heart failure syndromes

The **fundamental pathophysiological alteration** in acute heart failure syndromes is a **substantially and inappropriately elevated afterload** with a markedly elevated systemic resistance / markedly increased LV outflow impedance **exerting a high (end-)systolic load on the LV during ventricular ejection** [11, 20, 402].

This is referred to as afterload mismatch, defined by 'a fall in SV due to inappropriately high afterload' [403].

In **heart failure syndromes**, the **LV afterload** becomes the decisive determinant of cardiac performance [11–14]. As early as 1977 Cohn and Franciosa published their impressive diagram showing the correlation between afterload and cardiac performance/cardiac output (SV) (see Figure 1.6) [11].

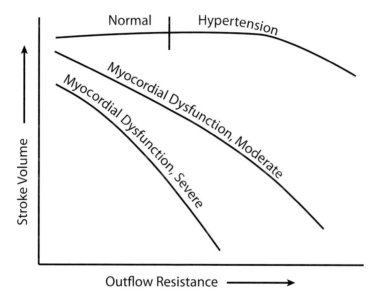

**Figure 1.6** Relation between SV(SW) and outflow resistance/impedance (adapted from Cohn, J. N. and Franciosa, J. A. [11]).

SV depends decisively on the magnitude of the afterload [3, 51, 102]. Furthermore, an elevated (after) load causes an increase in the LV filling pressure, producing high LVEDP [404] and thus affecting the already compromised diastolic properties of the heart, resulting in a further reduction of the LV filling rate [405, 406].

Afterload is inversely proportional to the stroke volume, **SV ~ 1/afterload** [402] and therefore an increase in afterload should result in a fall in SV and ejection fraction (EF) [370, 407]. However, in healthy hearts, despite an increase in wall tension due to the increased afterload, normal fibre shortening is accomplished by a compensatory increase in contractility [9, 102]. In the case of impaired LV function the increase in afterload is not tolerated, fibre length shortening is impaired, and a decrease in EF results [20].

The outcome of patients with Acute Heart Failure Syndromes correlates with the magnitude of LVEDP [17, 96, 97], and LVEDP correlates with the grade of activation of the sympathetic nervous system [408]. **Afterload mismatch** is the fundamental pathophysiological mechanism in acute heart failure [11, 20, 15, 402] and as such **afterload reduction** and thus a reduction in LVEDP is the treatment of choice [16, 17, 20], even in cases of low cardiac output (CO), as long as the MAP is appropriate ($\geq 70$–80 mm Hg) [409].

Finally, remember the following:
- afterload $\uparrow \rightarrow$ LVEDP $\uparrow$ [405, 406, 410–412],
- afterload $\uparrow \rightarrow$ LVESV $\uparrow$ [413] and SV $\downarrow$ [413] (In healthy persons SV may be maintained due to an increase in contractility.),
- afterload $\downarrow \rightarrow$ LVEDP $\downarrow$ [18, 19, 414] and LVEDD $\downarrow$ [18, 19, 102, 413, 414].
  Due to the law of LaPlace: When afterload $\downarrow \rightarrow$ LVEDP $\downarrow \rightarrow$ **diastolic** wall stress $\downarrow \rightarrow O_2$
  – requirement $\downarrow$ [21, 413] $\rightarrow$ LVEDD $\downarrow$ [18, 19, 102, 414],
- LV dilatation $\rightarrow$ wall stress $\uparrow \rightarrow$ afterload $\uparrow$ [368, 371],
- $\downarrow$ LVEDP $\rightarrow \downarrow$ afterload [100, 414] (this implication is inevitable and in accord with the law of LaPlace).

## 1.6    Contractility

### a)    Definition

Contractility is defined as the **inherent capacity of the myocardium to contract independently of changes in pre- and afterload** [415].

This capacity of **Intrinsic Force** of contraction is called **Contractility or Inotropy** [416, 417].

Braunwald writes, "Changes in cardiac performance independent of alterations in pre- and afterload are caused by 'contractility'. It has to be separated from changes in the performance due to a change in loading conditions" [415].

The sympathetic tone plays an important role in the regulation of contractility. The positive inotropic effect of increased sympathetic tone enables the heart, without a change in diastolic filling (without a change in the preload), to eject a higher SV or to maintain SV in case of increased afterload or increased resistance to ejection [418]. Kumar [9] found in healthy volunteers that the increase in SV due to volume loading is predominantly caused by an increase in contractility and only in minor part by the Frank-Starling mechanism, hence confirming previous results [155, 156]. Due to the increase in 'intrinsic' contractility, the end-systolic volume will decrease [9].

### b)    Measurement and quantification

It is very difficult to measure and to express contractility as a single, independent parameter. At the sarcomere level, contractility and load are interrelated; thus, they are not independent variables [419, 420]. Any parameter attempting to characterise 'true' contractility has to be independent of changes in pre- and afterload, LV-size and geometry and LV-pressure [421].

The rate of LV intraventricular pressure rise dp/dt, an index of the isovolumetric phase of the contraction [422], correlates well with the LV contractility [423]. The highest dp/dt, called dp/dt$_{max}$, throughout systole is expected to be proportional to the contractility [423]. Dp/dt$_{max}$, is sensitive of preload, but not of afterload because it is measured before the aortic valve opens [423].

Dp/dt$_{max}$ shows reasonably good sensitivity to detect and express changes in the 'true' inotropic status (intrinsic contractility) [424, 425]. It is the most valuable parameter to measure and express inotropy [424–428] and is currently the gold standard in representing the 'true' (intrinsic) contractility [429].

The contractile conditions of the ventricle are influenced by intrinsic properties of the ventricle at end-systole, the chamber elastance ($E_{es}$). These contractile properties of the ventricle can be quantified by the relationship between end-systolic left ventricular pressure (LVESP) and the end-systolic left ventricular volume (LVESV) [379, 391].

The ventricular pressure-volume relationship at end-systole is linear (at least under physiological conditions [430]) and its slope, $E_{es}$, **quantifies the ventricular (systolic) contractile properties** [379, 431, 432] (see part 9c of this chapter).

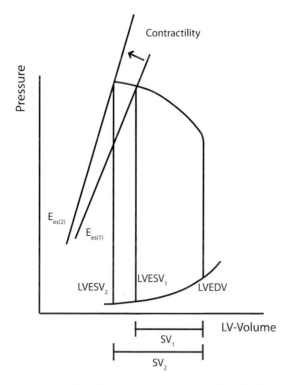

**Figure 1.7** The diagram depicts the effect of an increase in true contractility: The slope of $E_{es}$ becomes steeper, SV increases (SV2) and LVESV gets smaller (LVESV2). Thus, the improvement in contractility is reflected by a larger SV ejected, leading to a smaller LVESV while the LVEDV remains unchanged.

$E_{es}$ is defined as LVESP divided by LVESV, thus

$$E_{es} = \text{LVESP/LVESV} [433] = sBP \times 0.9/\text{LVESV}$$

$E_{es}$ is **roughly** load-independent [379], and Kass [434] found that over a wide range of load, $E_{es}$ is a powerful index of true LV-contractility [435–438].

When describing the systolic properties of the heart, we must differentiate between indices referring to the 'true' contractility and to other parameters describing the systolic function of the heart muscle or the heart performance. The latter two are less independent than the other indices and characterise the heart function in a more 'global' way. (For an overview see Baicu [398]).

**LV systolic performance** is characterised by the **stroke work**, taking into account that the heart has to generate pressure and flow (SV) [4, 102]:

$$\text{LV-SW} = \text{LV-SV} \times (\text{LVESP} - \text{LVEDP}) \times 0.0136 = \text{LV-SV} \times \text{MAP} \times 0.0136 \ [30, 439]$$

Normal values: 58–104 $\text{gm}^{-1}\text{m}^2$ [440, 441]

The systolic performance is influenced by load and ventricular configuration [442]; thus, it is not the same as contractility. Hence, abnormal performance may be present although contractility is normal (i.e. in case of high afterload) and vice versa, performance may be normal although the contractility is impaired (i.e. sepsis, MR) [442].

Whilst **cardiac work** describes the transferral of energy from the cardiac contraction to the development of blood flow [132], **cardiac power output** (CPO) describes the amount of energy generated by the heart that the whole systemic vasculature receives at the level of the aortic root [132]. Thus, it characterises the recruitable reserve still available in case of acute failure or shock in order to maintain the perfusion of the vital organs and hence reflects the severity of the patient's illness [132]. CPO has shown substantial prognostic power [132, 443] across the broad spectrum of acute heart failure syndromes and, in particular, in cardiogenic shock [132]. CPO is defined [132] as

$$\text{CPO} = \text{MAP} \times \text{CO}/451 \ (\text{Watts})$$

and follows the physical rules of fluids. Reflecting the essential task of the heart (to generate pressure and flow) [3, 4] CPO is a measure of cardiac pumping by coupling both pressure and flow domains [444].

Furthermore, CPO and its index, CPI, have shown superiority in determining the exact diagnosis of the actual heart failure syndrome compared to CI, BP, PCWP and their combination [15, 132]. Whilst the traditional haemodynamic measures and their presumed target values used in treatment protocols have been misleading [445] they have also failed to show any relevant effect when therapy was titrated due to their values [446].

CPO appears to be a better parameter than CPI for predicting outcome. Adjustment of CPO for body size, yielding CPI, showed a weaker association with mortality [447–449]. A CPO ≤ 0.53 most accurately predicts a high likelihood of in-hospital mortality [132, 443].

Conventionally SVI and SWI were used as powerful predictors of short term mortality in cardiogenic shock complicating AMI [450], but the use of CPO is now thought preferable.

The **LV systolic function** of the heart can be described in a number of ways but, **ejection fraction** (EF, %) is still the most frequently used parameter. EF is determined by the interaction of arterial and ventricular properties and is dependent on the afterload, and thus it is not exclusively governed by the LV [389, 400, 451].

$$EF\% = [(LVEDV - LVESV)/LVEDV] \times 100;$$
$$EF\% = SV/LVEDV \text{ [452, 453].}$$

However,

$$\text{afterload} \uparrow \rightarrow EF \downarrow \text{ and vice versa [370, 407].}$$

EF is thus far from being an ideal parameter to assess contractility. EF depends on afterload as well as on preload and heart volume or mass [402, 425, 454, 455].
   EF will fail to report:
- excess afterload (EF reduced although the contractility is normal) [456],
- in case of augmented preload (i.e. MR), EF will overestimate the systolic function, missing myocardial dysfunction [457, 458],
- in concentric LV-H, EF measurement signals normal systolic function, although substantial dysfunction may be present [459].

Normal values EF > 55% [452, 453, 460–466]; an EF > 40% is considered reasonable [460–468].
   Despite its shortcomings, Braunwald [442] and Gillebert [469] state that EF is the best parameter to describe overall contractility in comparison to all others currently in use.

'True' **LV-contractility** is best expressed by:
- $dp/dt_{max}$     (mm Hg/s), normal values 1400–2200 [470]
- $E_{es}$          (mm Hg/ml), normal value about 2.0 [400, 471].
$E_{es}$ <1 mm Hg/ml is found in dilated and failing hearts [472], in case of hypertrophy there will be a significant increase – up to 4 mm Hg/ml [473].
   It has to be stressed that CI is not an index of contractility, but rather a measure of cardiovascular flow: CI is affected by contractility, vascular stiffness and resistance, intravascular volume and filling pressures [132]. Furthermore, there is no normal CO/CI, since metabolic demands can vary widely [119].

## c)    **Inotropic medications**

Medications able to increase the myocardial contractility are called **inotropes**. In recent years the administration of inotropic drugs has been overshadowed by clear and growing evidence of adverse events and **increased mortality** [151, 474–478], particularly when given in patients with reasonably preserved left ventricular function (EF > 40%) [479, 480]. Conners [481] and

Sandham [482] found a significantly **increased mortality when clinically stable patients** were treated with conventional inotropic agents secondary to numerically low cardiac output. Only patients who absolutely require inotropic support secondary to low output as result of severely impaired **contractility and** who are **resistant** to other treatments should be treated by such drugs [467, 483].

The European Society of Cardiology (ESC) recommends inotropic agents in heart failure syndromes if the illness has deteriorated to become life-threatening and the situation has become critically dependent on the haemodynamics: "Inotropic agents are indicated in the presence of peripheral hypoperfusion with or without congestion or pulmonary oedema **refractory** to diuretics and **vasodilators** at optimal dosages" [467].

The relatively newly developed drug **Levosimendan**, a calcium-sensitising and vasodilating agent [484, 485] has shown very encouraging effects and results in the treatment of severe heart failure [486–491] and cardiogenic shock [492]. Although the recently finished REVIVE-2 [493] and SURVIVE study [494] could not confirm a better outcome in the levosimendan group compared to those patients treated with dobutamine, levosimendan seems nevertheless to be the more favourable drug compared with dobutamine in regard to both pharmacological effects and outcome (less mortality) as reported previously in several studies [487, 489, 490, 495, 496]. Even in the SURVIVE study [494], patients admitted with an acute exacerbation of chronic heart failure or patients on beta-blockers due to chronic heart failure and who acutely decompensated showed a significant decrease in mortality when treated with levosimendan rather than dobutamine [497].

Levosimendan intervenes more 'physiologically' on the impaired contractility. The reduced myofilamental responsiveness to calcium is a major determinant of systolic myocardial depression [498]. Levosimendan augments the calcium sensitivity without increasing the intracellular calcium-concentration [499].

## 1.7    Heart rate and contractility

At the end of the 19th century Bowditch published his observation that the force of heart contraction increases – up to a limit – with an increase in heart rate [417].

The peak isometric force increases with increasing heart rate [417, 500]. This is due to the fact that calcium will accumulate within the myocytes when diastole shortens [501] (which happens with increasing heart rate). In the case of a compromised or failing heart this effect is attenuated, or even the opposite may happen – with increasing heart rate the force of contraction will decrease [500, 502, 503]. When the tachycardia exceeds 130/min, the severity of myocardial impairment correlates with the extent of tachycardia [504]. Furthermore, tachycardia will always precede a fall in BP [323].

Thus, in the **case of tachycardia** in a compromised heart the **reduction in heart rate** will **increase the cardiac contraction and hence SV** (MAP and organ perfusion):

$$\text{Heart rate} \downarrow \rightarrow \uparrow \text{EF [505].}$$

In heart failure patients developing or suffering from atrial fibrillation, a heart rate of 100–110/min is acceptable [506].

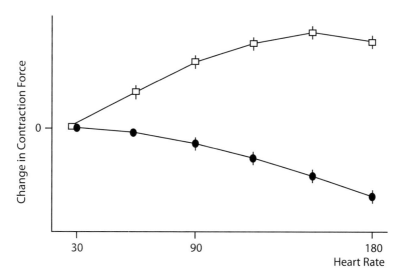

**Figure 1.8** Adapted from Bowditch [417], copied from Böhm, M, *Herzinsuffizienz*, chapter 4, Thieme Verlag, 2000, p. 29.

## 1.8    Diastolic ventricular interaction (DVI)

### a)    Definition

Sharing the interventricular septum and being enclosed by the "same" pericardium, **interactions between the right and left ventricle** occur [27, 507–509]. This interaction functionally mainly occurs in diastole and is therefore called the **diastolic ventricular interaction (DVI)**, although it was previously known as interventricular interdependence.

DVI describes the direct influence of changes in volume of one ventricle on the other [27] or, more fully, taking all possible involved parameters into account, the influence on the compliance [510] of one ventricle by changes in volume, intraventricular pressure and compliance (or a combination) of the other ventricle [27, 507, 508, 511–514]. In particular, **acute** changes in the conditions will influence the other ventricle more dramatically [27, 45, 52, 515].

These diastolic interactions are mediated via the shared structures of the two ventricles, the interventricular septum and the pericardium. The pericardium has constraining effects on ventricular filling due to its poor distensibility and its pressure transmitting effects [52, 54, 516]. The interaction mediated by the septum and the pericardium is called '**direct**' interaction, while the so called '**series**' interaction refers simply to the physical relation between the two ventricles and their outputs: The two ventricles are coupled in a row, one after the other and thus the output necessarily has to be equal over time [37, 45].

## b)    Septum and trans-septal pressure

The shape of the septum, under physiological conditions, is concave when viewed from the LV side. There is no difference during systole and diastole, due to the fact that the LVEDP always remains higher than the RVEDP and increases proportionately during systole [45]. Kingma established proof that the position of the septum is determined by the end-diastolic pressure gradient between LV and RV [517]:

$$\text{Transseptal pressure gradient} = \text{LVEDP} - \text{RVEDP [517].}$$

In disease, the position of the septum can change markedly due to changes in the pressure gradient, which will alter the end-diastolic volumes substantially [52–54, 120, 517–519]. In acute RV pressure or volume overload Kingma showed that the interventricular septum becomes flattened or even convex at end-diastole due to RV dilatation and raised RVEDP, diminishing the transseptal pressure gradient and pushing the septum towards the left ventricle [517]. Numerous publications confirm the change in the septum position in different diseases such as acute and chronic pulmonary hypertension [52–54, 512, 520], congestive heart failure [26, 27], and mechanical ventilation [120].

This leftward shift of the septum contributes significantly to the reduction in LV-filling; thus, total LV-volume and end-diastolic volume are reduced and the SV will fall as a consequence.

The very poorly distensible pericardium supports this process by exerting constraint, restricting the total heart volume from changing [519, 521].

## c)    Pericardium

All cardiac chambers (except the posterior part of the LA where the pulmonary veins enter) are enclosed by the pericardium. It works as a tight, unyielding band around the minor axis of the heart, fixing the cross sectional area of the heart and causing direct ventricular interaction [522].

Thus, an **increase in the cross-sectional area of one ventricle**, i.e. due to volume loading or enlargement, necessarily **reduces the area of the opposite ventricle** with less filling potential, **causing an increase in the pericardial pressure**, and **altering the transmural pressure** [26, 522]. The total cardiac volume remains **unchanged** [519, 521].

Increasing pressures in the pericardial space will exert a progressive restraining effect on ventricular filling, termed **pericardial constraint** [519]. When the pericardium becomes stretched due to enlargement of the ventricles, such as in chronic heart failure or due to volume loading, the filling – in particular the left ventricular filling – becomes significantly restrained [26, 131]. With further stretch the pericardium is even less distensible [516] and, **especially in cases of acute change,** the pericardium, with its constraining effect, plays a key role in loading conditions [94, 508, 523, 524]. Under those conditions the pericardial pressure (PP) will increase progressively and will significantly constrain the filling. PP rises in an exponential manner [522] and once the pericardium becomes 'overstretched', an exponential increase in LVEDP is seen [91, 525].

Raised intra-thoracic pressure, i.e. due to raised intra-abdominal pressure, chest infection, etc., will affect, secondary to an increased constraint on the thin walled RV, the RVEDP more than the LVEDP (rise in RVEDP > rise in LVEDP) [52, 53]. Hence, the transmural LVEDP (= LVEDP − RAP/CVP; see part 3b of this chapter) will decrease with less LVEDV and less LV end-diastolic fibre stretch, and a reduced SV will result.

Ventricular interaction due to pericardial constraint is diminished as long as the PP is < 5 mm Hg [130]; when exceeding 9–10 mm Hg the pericardium will exert a significant constraint on ventricular filling [71, 131]. Furthermore, when intraventricular LVEDP exceeds 10(12)–15 mm Hg, the LVEDP-LVEDV relation becomes much steeper and the pericardium limits further increases in LV volume [91, 173, 525].

## d)      Pulmonary hypertension and the risk of DVI

In **pulmonary hypertension** fluid administration is shown to increase RVEDP more than LVEDP [52, 53]. The concomitant (along with RVEDP) increase in pericardial pressure will exceed the rise of the LVEDP (due to a higher increase of RVEDP compared with LVEDP),

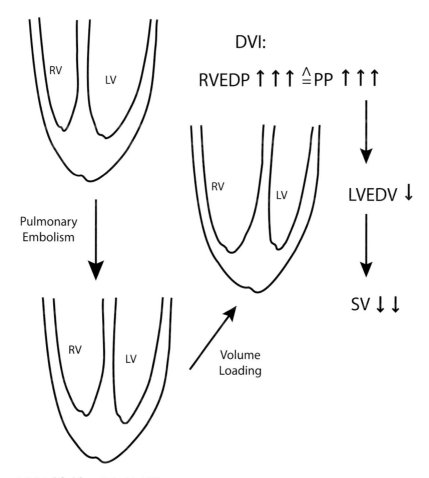

**Figure 1.9** Modified from Belenkie [45].

thus transmural LVEDP and therefore LV-preload will be reduced due to pericardial constraint [26, 57].

**Fluid administration in pulmonary hypertension**

→ ↑ RVEDP > ↑ LVEDP (more constraint on RV), and
   ↑ PP > ↑ intraventricular LVEDP
→ transmural LVEDP ↓ and thus LVEDV ↓ [30, 26, 46] with consecutive ↓ **LV-SV** [42, 43].

(An additional effect will be exerted by the leftward shift of the septum, reducing the LV-area and thus the LVEDV [52–54, 512, 520]).

## e)    Acutely exacerbated chronic congestive (left-sided or biventricular) heart failure

An acute exacerbation of chronic congestive heart failure is often crucial in the disease's course and may be the final point in a critical illness [526–528]. In this situation, **DVI** may have a substantial impact on the haemodynamics and has to be taken into the therapeutic considerations [52, 53, 529–531].

A sudden rise in RV-afterload / increase in RV-outflow impedance and/or a loss in contractility, i.e. due to acute RV myocardial infarction [532, 533], will always induce RV dilatation [534–537], a fall in RV-EF [535, 536] and a substantial increase in RVEDP [76, 368, 538]. This implies a considerable rise in PP and a leftward shift of the septum, which compromises LV filling [26, 30, 46, 49, 60, 62, 63, 71, 517, 519, 521].

**Acute ↑ RV-outflow impedance / RV-afterload**
↓
RV-dilatation (RVEDD ↑), ↑ RVEDP, and ↓ RV-EF
↓ **DVI** [52, 53, 529–531]
↓ transmural LVEDP → ↓ **LV-SV** (LV-SW) [26, 30, 46] / ↓ **blood pressure.**

Atherton [27] showed that, in patients with **chronic congestive heart failure and high LVEDP** (pulmonary hypertension), LV-filling was markedly impeded due to direct diastolic inter-ventricular interaction via the septum and from the stretched pericardium (pericardial constraint): Volume **un**loading resulted, as expected, in reduction of the RVEDV, but LVEDV "paradoxically" increased.

In nearly 50% of all patients suffering from congestive HF, pericardial constraint plays a marked role [27] and unloading leads to an improvement in cardiac performance. Even if there is less pericardial constraint present, as in the other 50% of patients studied by Atherton, the reduction in LVEDV secondary to volume unloading did not significantly compromise the haemodynamic situation.

These results are consistent with the findings by Dupuis, who showed that a reduction in PCWP in patients with congestive HF resulted in an increased SV and SW even though LVEDP

fell [55]. Stevenson established in 1986 that volume unloading in patients with severe congestive heart failure and high filling pressures showed clear beneficial results, with an improvement
in clinical short and long term outcome [73].

Moore explored the underlying pathophysiological mechanisms and established our current
therapeutic approach [26]. In patients with congestive HF, and thus secondary pulmonary
hypertension, direct diastolic ventricular interaction plays a substantial role in the LV-dysfunction responsible for the reduced LV-SV. The common approach of administering volume to a
patient with low blood pressure will, in acutely decompensated chronic heart failure, worsen the
haemodynamic and clinical situation [26]. Volume **unloading** will stabilise the situation.

**Pathophysiology** of chronic congestive HF:

$$\textbf{LV is enlarged, LVEDP} \uparrow \text{ (often high)} \quad \rightarrow \textbf{RVEDP} \uparrow - \uparrow\uparrow$$
$$\rightarrow \text{RVEDV/RVEDD} \uparrow$$

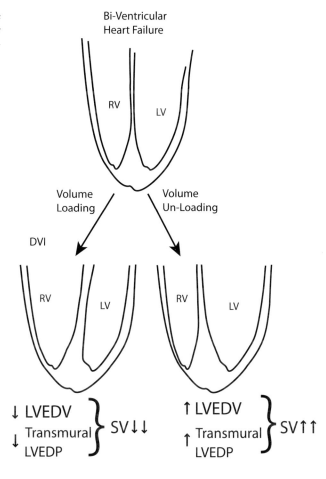

**Figure 1.10**  Diagram to show the position of the interventricular septum in different loading conditions.

The **elevation of the RVEDP** is either due to **pericardial constraint** [26, 27] following the rule of total cardiac volume [519, 521] and/or due to (chronically) ↑ **RV-afterload** (pulmonary hypertension caused by ↑ LVEDP) [534, 535, 539–541]. Furthermore, an elevated RV-afterload / elevated RV outflow impedance, as found in pulmonary hypertension due to a raised LVEDP, will always induce RV enlargement, hence ↑ RVEDD and ↑ RVEDV [534–537].

Additionally, the ↑ in transseptal pressure gradient as a consequence of raised LVEDP/ LVEDV in LV failure pushes the septum towards the right ventricle, though RVEDP will ↑ [26, 27, 517]. This will **even be present** in the case of a 'relatively low LVEDP when the LV is very compliant [517].

Thus: ↑/↑↑↑ in RVEDP, and the ↑/↑↑↑ in RVEDD and RVEDV → parallel ↑/↑↑↑ PP [49, 62, 63, 66, 71].

If volume is given in this situation:

**Volume loading** → further ↑ RVEDP (with ↑ **RVEDP** >↑ **LVEDP** [52, 53])    →
　　　　　　　　　↑ in RVEDD due to ↑ RVEDV and (further) ↑ PP
　　　　　　　　　　　　　　　　　↓

1. transseptal pressure gradient now ↓ [517], and hence leftward shift of the septum → reduced LV-filling (constant total cardiac volume [519, 521])    → LV-SV ↓ [42, 43].

2. due to a parallel rise of PP with RVEDP [49, 62, 63, 66, 71], the pericardial constraint will increasingly impede LV filling: transmural-LVEDP ↓ → LVEDV ↓ [26, 30, 41, 46] → LV-SV ↓ [42, 43].

Unloading is the treatment of choice (GTN, diuretics):

**Volume unloading** → RVEDP ↓, RVEDV ↓ and LVEDP ↓ [26, 27, 55]
　　　　　　　　　　(but LVEDP ↓ < RVEDP ↓ [52,53]),
　　　　　　　PP ↓ (equal and parallel to RVEDP) [49, 66, 71]
　　　　　　　　　　　↓

1. Transseptal pressure gradient ↑ [517], hence septum shifts to the right → **LV-area** ↑ (LVEDD ↑) → LVEDV ↑    → LV-SV ↑ [42, 43].

2. Less pericardial constraint of the left ventricle due to ↓ PP transmural LVEDP ↑ [26, 27, 41, 55] → LVEDV ↑ [26, 27, 30, 46, 55]    → LV-SV ↑ [42, 43].

Although the heart is unloaded, the SV increases: This is often called the 'paradoxical ↑' in SV.

A simplified summary of the unloading process [27]:

**RV-preload** ↓ → RVEDV ↓ → RVEDD ↓ → LVEDD ↑ → LVEDV ↑ → LV-SV ↑/BP ↑

It is important to remember that evidence of haemodynamically significant DVI was found in 50% of all patients with congestive HF, and even if a relevant DVI is not present, unloading reduced the LVEDV only marginally and did not compromise the haemodynamic situation (no fall in blood pressure) [26–28, 46, 55]. Hence, all patients with acutely decompensated chronic congestive heart failure should be treated by volume unloading.

## f)    Conclusions

Ventricular interaction has a considerable impact on the haemodynamic situation, particularly in critically ill patients with circulatory compromise [30, 52, 182, 542, 543]. Circumstances **suggestive of significant DVI** are the **combination of pulmonary hypertension (PH) and elevated CVP**, especially in right-sided heart dysfunction/failure, which always implies increased PP [30].

Examples are:
- **acute pulmonary embolism** [52, 54],
- **acute right HF** ( RV-AMI, ARDS, sepsis) [46, 282, 539],
- **exacerbation of chronic RV-dysfunction** (COPD with acute exacerbation) [53],
- **acutely exacerbated chronic congestive HF** [26, 27, 55, 539, 541] **with enlarged LV, particularly in cases where the LVEDP is high** [26, 27, 55],
- **intubation and mechanical ventilation, in particular in patients with acute/chronic pulmonary hypertension** [53, 120, 179],
- **PEEP** effects the heart in the same way as (cardiac) tamponade [192]; when PEEP >12 mm $H_2O$, an RV-pressure load (RVEDP ↑) and a septum shift was found [544],
- **other causes of a considerably increased intra-thoracic pressure** [77] such as severe chest infection, tension pneumothorax [62] and **increased intra-abdominal pressure** [78] as in severe abdominal infection, ascites or abdominal compartment syndrome.

All of the above will have an impact on the potential therapy and consideration of these should change our daily practice markedly [26, 28, 46, 52, 515, 545].

Volume loading can no longer be recommended in acute RV dysfunction/RV-failure [52, 91, 130, 546–551] and volume loading due to low blood pressure in acutely decompensated congestive heart failure carries a very high risk of worsening the situation and, as such, unloading is the approach of choice [26, 27, 46, 55, 151, 552, 553].

## 1.9    Ventriculo-arterial coupling

## a)    Definition

**Ventricular-arterial coupling** is the interaction between ventricular and arterial system and describes the transmission of the ventricular performance to the systemic circulation [554]. It is an important determinant of cardiac performance [386, 389, 451]. Starling demands that the evaluation of the LV performance should only be done in the context of its interaction with the systemic arterial system [555] – a requirement proposed elsewhere as well [11, 15, 552, 556, 557]. **The systolic function can only be evaluated in light of the afterload** which the ventricle faces during systole [15, 132, 398, 467].

The heart has to generate **flow and pressure** to ensure an adequate output [4, 102]. The net **flow and pressure output** developed by the heart as a pump depends upon [102]:

- intrinsic properties of the heart (end-diastolic and end-systolic chamber stiffness),
- properties of the blood – contribute to the arterial load,
- arterial properties (arterial load) comprising arterial compliance, characteristic aortic impedance, SVR, and the pulsatile component (in particular wave reflections) of the vessel system.

Vascular and ventricular properties have to match in order to achieve a maximal, efficient transfer of mechanical energy aiming for maximal SW [391, 555, 558–561].

Studies by Piene [562] and by Piene and Sund [248] have established that the work of the heart and the interaction of the ventricle with the arterial system can be calculated from the **ventricular pressure-volume – time relationship and the load impedance** [248, 562].

## b)  Arterial elastance

The **characterisation of the vascular load** faced by the ventricle during systole is best described by the **effective arterial elastance ($E_a$)** [389, 390, 561]. It was K. Sunagawa [389] who 'distilled' the vascular impedance into the 'effective' arterial elastance (characterising the arterial pressure measured in the arterial system at any given ejected SV [386] which can easily be coupled with ventricular pressure-volume loops and relations [563]). The effective arterial elastance incorporates the principle elements of the vascular load [391, 564] as:

- peripheral resistance,
- total lumped vascular compliance,
- characteristic impedance, and
- systolic and diastolic time intervals.

Hence, "$E_a$ combines various aspects of the total arterial input impedance into effective stiffness" dominated by arterial resistance as the primary component of impedance load [386]. The advantage of impedance as a descriptor of hydraulic load (vascular load) is that it characterises the properties of the vessel bed **independently from cardiac output** [392–394]. Furthermore, $E_a$ has been shown to reflect aspects of the ventricular-arterial interaction [364, 393] and so is a coupling parameter as well [364].

## c)  Ventricular elastance

The mechanical energy of ventricular contraction is transferred to the blood within the chamber, providing it with hydraulic energy [565, 566] to face the impedance of the vascular system (the arterial load) and enabling the heart to overcome those afterloaded forces [15, 395, 398, 567].

**The power of output and the stroke work generated** depend on:

- preload (preload dependent recruitable SW/SV – described by the law of Frank [42] and Starling [43]),
- input impedance of the arterial system $E_a$ [389, 559, 567],
- **intrinsic properties of the ventricle at end-systole**, the so-called **chamber elastance ($E_{es}$)** [431, 432, 568, 569].

The **intrinsic ventricular properties at end-systole** are scientifically depicted by the pressure-volume relation [379, 391]. The **slope of ventricular pressure-volume relationship at end-systole, $E_{es}$**, quantifies the ventricular contractile properties [379, 431, 432]. The ventricular compliance is the inverse of elastance [570].

An $E_{es}$ (= LVESP/LVESV [433], normal value ~ 2.0 mm Hg/ml [400, 471] ) of < 1.0 mm Hg/ml is found in dilated and failing hearts [472] whereas an $E_{es}$ > 3–4 mm Hg/ml is found in hypertrophied hearts [473].

**Abnormal end-systolic ventricular stiffness** is a **characteristic** finding in **diastolic dysfunction** [571–575] and **increased left ventricular stiffness** makes the patient **vulnerable to developing pulmonary oedema** [575].

## d)   Ventriculo-arterial coupling

The $E_a/E_{es}$ **ratio** describes the coupling of the ventricular and arterial system. $E_a/E_{es}$ is a predictor of the efficiency of the energy transfer from the ventricle to the vascular system [576] and reflects the matching of cardiac systolic and arterial properties [472].

As a rule, a decrease in $E_a$ will lead to an increase in $E_{es}$ [396] and vice versa [554]. The $E_a/E_{es}$ ratio is a useful parameter in order to characterise the LV-pump function under varying loading and inotropic conditions [391, 555, 577].

Furthermore,

$$E_a/E_{es} \sim 1/EF \ [578]$$

(assuming the intercept volume (Vo) is zero or nearly zero, which is not the case in dilated hearts [364]).

The $E_a/E_{es}$ ratio provides information about:

- overall systolic LV-function,
- max. LV-SV (SW), and
- mechanical efficiency of the LV-pump [555, 578]

The normal ratio of $E_a/E_{es}$ = 0.6 to 1.2 [396, 555, 571]. An $E_a/E_{es} \geq 2$ reflects, in general, a depressed LV inotropic state ($E_{es} \downarrow$) coupled with high vascular resistance ($E_a \uparrow$) [472, 571].

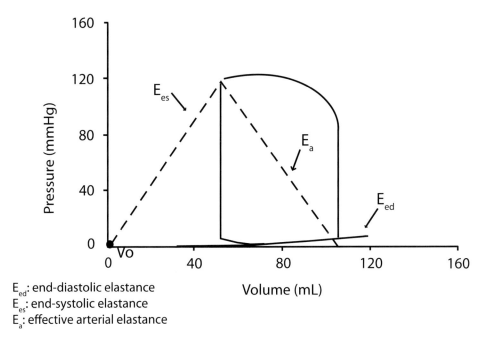

$E_{ed}$: end-diastolic elastance
$E_{es}$: end-systolic elastance
$E_{a}$: effective arterial elastance

**Figure 1.11** Modified from Kass [386].

### e)        Deranged coupling

With aging and in diseases such as hypertension, $E_a$ increases [400, 411, 471, 579]. An increase in $E_a$ is accompanied by an increase in $E_{es}$ due to a rise in ventricular stiffness [400, 471, 580, 581]: The diastolic cardiac function is affected by the arterial compliance and an increase in vascular stiffness will lead to a concomitant reduction in ventricular compliance [471]. As described above, $E_a$ and $E_{es}$ have to match in order to achieve optimal energy transfer and mechanical efficiency; thus, the increase in $E_{es}$ may be seen as a necessary adaption in order to match the vascular properties [400, 555, 571].

On the other hand, $E_{es}$ is known to be pathologically high in diastolic dysfunction [471, 571–575, 582] and specific myocardial diseases such as amyloidosis [583].

However, these circumstances may lead to adverse or deranged **coupling**, where $E_a$ and $E_{es}$ do not match and the transfer of energy from myocardium to vasculature becomes inefficient. In the case of impaired LV compliance, as in diastolic dysfunction, adverse coupling may allow a rise in afterload (i.e. increasing blood pressure, increase in circulating volume) to cause a **disproportionate** increase in $E_{es}$ and $E_a$ (increase $E_{es}$ > increase $E_a$) [400, 471]. Furthermore, LV stiffness in the presence of vascular stiffening is shown to amplify the impact of even small increases in LV-filling on cardiac workload and arterial pressure reflected by a disproportional increase in sBP for any relative change in LVEDV [391, 400]. Severe consequences may result: Najjer [584] concluded that an acute rise in $E_a$, but with an otherwise normal arterial elastance, might induce a substantial increase in LVEDP in the elderly with higher $E_{es}$ (age-related). Hundley showed that a reduced aortic distensibility ($E_a \uparrow$) can cause (acute) heart failure [411] and

**Figure 1.12** Secondary to a rise in afterload (BP ↑), the $E_{es}$ of 5.6 measured in HFNEF increased by 145% (compared to normal controls) while the $E_a$ increased by just 33% (adapted from Kawaguchi [471]).

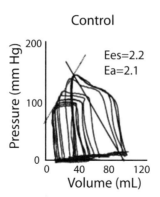

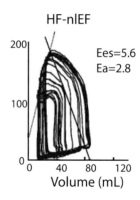

Kawaguchi [471] established further substantial evidence that arterial stiffening when combined with ventricular stiffness (attributed to age, hypertension and/or diastolic dysfunction) can lead to pulmonary oedema [585, 586]. This condition can occur when **deranged coupling** causes a **marked rise in the systolic LV-load** secondary to acutely altered afterload [471]. The increase in systolic load induces a **prolongation of the diastolic LV-relaxation** [412, 587] and **compromises LV-filling** [412]; the latter both induce a substantial increase in LVEDP [412, 571] which may lead to decompensation and pulmonary oedema [585, 586].

Therefore, **acute changes in afterload** along with deranged ventriculo-arterial coupling producing a disproportionate transmission of vascular stiffening onto the ventricle [471] can increase the LVEDP markedly [400, 412, 582]. Hence, **flash pulmonary oedema** may be seen as a vascular, rather than a purely cardiac disorder [471, 582].

(This pathophysiology is quite different from that underlying pulmonary oedema in congestive heart failure, where it usually develops relatively 'slowly' due to (severe) fluid overload [588]).

If a rapid rise in afterload is the underlying pathophysiological mechanism causing pulmonary oedema, vasodilators have to be the preferred therapy [589]; whilst in fluid overload, diuretics (low to moderate dose) are the drug of choice.

## 1.10 Evaluation and assessment of the cardiac performance

As described previously the heart has to generate pressure and flow in order to pump the blood into the vasculature and hence ensure sufficient circulation [102, 590, 591]. Parameters currently used to measure cardiac (systolic) performance are the CPO and SW (see part 6 of this chapter) [132, 439–441, 444, 450]. Both parameters integrate the fundamental cardiac functions [4, 15, 102, 132, 450]. In comparison to SW, CPO characterises the recruitable reserve still available in cases of acute failure and in shock, which may be utilised to maintain the perfusion of the vital organs and hence reflects the severity of the patient's illness [132].

It should be noted that SV/SVI or even CO/CI do not reflect the cardiac pump function. They do not incorporate the pressure generation, nor are they an index of contractility. SVI/CI is affected by contractility, vascular stiffness and resistance, intravascular volume, and filling pressures [132]. CI is insufficient for accurate diagnosis and treatment titration in acute heart failure [245, 446, 592, 593]. Furthermore, there is no normal range for CO/CI, since metabolic demands can vary widely [119].

Flow represented by SV(CO) is dependent on afterload [3, 51, 104]. In particular, in acutely compromised heart function (either due to impaired contractility and/or due to abnormal loading conditions) there is plenty of evidence that afterload is the most important determinate of pump function [11–15]. Cotter [15] established proof that the accurate diagnosis of the different heart failure syndromes can only be made when coupling both cardiac pumping abilities and afterload. He provided strong evidence that the cardiac pump ability can only be assessed correctly if related to the afterload present at the same moment as the pump function is measured [15].

Cotter's results have been validated and confirmed in several large studies covering a broad spectrum of primary cardiac diseases [132, 443]. Additionally, CPO (CPI) has substantial evidence supporting it as a powerful and robust prognostic parameter [15, 132, 443] (see part 6 of this chapter as well as Chapter 2).

The relationship between (simultaneously) measured/calculated CPI and afterload (repre-

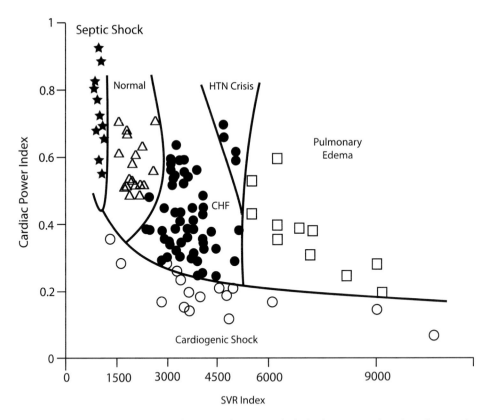

**Figure 1.13** Relationship between cardiac pump function and afterload in various clinical conditions. Abbreviations: CHF – acute congestive heart failure; HTN crisis – hypertensive crisis; CPI-cardiac power index, CPI = MAP × CI × 0.0022; SVRI – systemic vascular resistance index, SVRI = (MAP-RA): CI); (adapted from Cotter [15]).

sented by SVRI) has been shown to provide pivotal information about the actual haemodynamic situation (appropriate SVRI or inappropriately high/low [15]) and gives decisive information on the best management strategy [15, 132, 450].

In the special case of septic shock, an inverse correlation between cardiac performance and afterload has been demonstrated [594]. Furthermore, Müller-Werdan [595] demonstrated that septic cardiomyopathy is characterised by a significantly reduced cardiac performance which is relative to the effective afterload. Again, the actual cardiac pump function in relation to the afterload present provides strong prognostic information as well as clues on how to treat the patient (e.g. the timing of when inotropic support may be indicated) [596, 597].

Although quite clearly having disadvantages and limitations in sensitivity and accuracy of reflecting the LV load at end-systole, the afterload [370, 385] is still well represented by the SVR/SVRI, which accounts for 95% of the resistance to ejection (arterial resistance is the dominant component of impedance load) [363, 386]. Furthermore, SVR may be very helpful in clarifying the diagnosis [15, 132, 363], particularly in hypotensive patients [15, 132].

In summary, **cardiac pump function** can (and should) only be **accurately and reliably evaluated** in **relation to the actual afterload** [11–13, 15, 132, 286, 299, 443, 595–599]. At the sarcomere level, contractility and load are interrelated and thus not independent variables [419, 420]. Furthermore, the consideration of the pump function in the light of the afterload will give substantial information about the severity of the patient's situation, the mortality, and the appropriate therapeutic approach [15, 132, 443, 595, 596, 600]. Figure 1.13 depicts the fundamental relationship between cardiac pump function and afterload in various clinical conditions – a very practical approach to classify and diagnose patients as well as adding substantial information to the prognosis and therapy.

## 1.11  Summary

### a) Key physiology

Frank [42] and Starling [43] established proof that, with increasing fibre length, the force of contraction will increase and so will the ventricular stroke volume. The pressure exerted on the myocardial fibres, the so-called effective distending pressure or '**transmural**' **LVEDP**, is the intra-cavitary LVEDP (commonly just called LVEDP) minus the **surrounding pressure(s)** [41]:

Transmural LVEDP = LVEDP – surrounding pressure = PCWP – RA = PCWP – CVP

(with CVP reflecting the surrounding pressure [26, 59, 62, 64–66]).

An **increase in SV** subsequent to an increase in preload (higher LVEDV) **depends** not only on the change in the left ventricular **filling** but on the **contractile** capabilities (myocardial responsiveness) as well [9], particularly in the case of compromised cardiac function [10, 82, 100]. SV is determined by venous return **and** cardiac performance (afterload, heart rate and in particular contractility) [37–39].

**Cardiac (pump) function**, represented by CPO/CPI or SW, **can only be evaluated in relation to afterload** [12, 13, 15, 132, 299, 443, 598] and the original diagram by Cotter [15] gives a good approach to diagnosis, therapy, and treatment in daily practice.

## b)     Afterload

The fundamental pathophysiological alteration of acute heart failure syndromes is an **afterload mismatch** with a markedly elevated resistance / high input impedance (high end-systolic wall stress) during ventricular ejection [11, 20, 402].

The **LV afterload** becomes the **decisive determinant of cardiac performance** [11–14]; thus, cardiac performance can only be assessed in light of the actual afterload [15, 132]. SV becomes dependent on the afterload [3, 51, 102] with SV ~ 1/afterload [36, 402].

## c)     Systolic function

EF, as an index of the global **systolic function** [389, 400], is the most frequently used parameter to estimate systolic performance, and gives an impression of contractility. However,

$$\text{afterload} \uparrow \rightarrow \text{EF} \downarrow \text{ and vice versa [370, 407].}$$

EF may overestimate the systolic function in cases of excess afterload (EF reduced although the contractility is normal) [456] and augmented preload (i.e. MR). EF may miss myocardial dysfunction [457, 458] in concentric LV-hypertrophy; EF may signal normal systolic function, although substantial dysfunction may be present [459].

## d)     Volume status

It is crucial to evaluate the actual fluid status of the central cardiovascular system and the most likely response to volume expansion. An assessment of the dynamic indices such as LV stroke volume variation (SV-V) [10, 125, 267] peripherally or centrally, systolic BP-variation (SP-V) [208] or pulse pressure variation (PP-V) [125], is highly advisable [126, 161, 162, 172, 178, 180, 181]. The dynamic parameters reflect changes in LV-SV due to heart-lung interactions induced by mechanical ventilation [125, 125, 147, 177, 182–185].

Blind volume administration [134], with its potential risk of fluid overload, may increase patient mortality [233–236, 268], but in life-threatening situations with severe hypotension and tissue hypoperfusion, even without basic monitoring or central blood flow measurements, a fluid challenge as described by Vincent and Weil [137] is justifiable [245].

Use the **CVP** as:
- an index of PP [59, 62–66] and indicator of possible **DVI** [30], particularly when CVP is > 9–10 mm Hg [49, 71, 130] or if increase by > 5 mm Hg due to volume loading [137],
- a marker of cardiovascular dysfunction if elevated (> 7–8 mm Hg) [119], especially as an indicator of right heart dysfunction/failure [118], if clinically suspected and CVP ≥ 9–10 mm Hg [30, 546, 547].

Use **EVLW(I)** as:
- an index of fluid overload [250, 259, 260] and to guide fluid therapy [249–251],
- an indicator of (early) cardiogenic (hydrostatic) pulmonary oedema [145, 250, 264],

- a **very strong prognostic index implicating,** as a rule, **absolute fluid restriction if elevated**
(EVLWI > 10 ml/kg) [233–235, 249, 268].

The derived PVPI is a very helpful tool to differentiate non-cardiogenic pulmonary oedema (PVPI ≥ 3 [238]) from cardiogenic pulmonary oedema (PVPI 1–3)[254, 234, 235, 261] and/or to identify a significant capillary leakage (PVPI = EVLW/PBV) [238, 254, 261, 262].

## e)    Ventriculo-arterial coupling

Acute changes in afterload along with deranged ventriculo-arterial coupling produce a disproportionate transmission of vascular stiffening onto the ventricle [471], which can increase the LVEDP markedly [400, 412, 582]. Flash pulmonary oedema may occur despite normal systolic function [411, 471, 582] and may be regarded as a vascular, rather than a purely cardiac, disorder [601, 602].

## f)    DVI

DVI has a considerable impact on the haemodynamics. Significant DVI is suggested by a combination of PH and elevated CVP, especially in case of RV-dysfunction/failure [46, 52–55, 77, 78, 192]. In acute exacerbations of chronic congestive heart failure, in particular if LVEDP is elevated, due to DVI, volume unloading will lead to a 'paradoxial' increase in LV-SV and is thus the treatment of choice [26, 27, 55, 73]. Even if the patient is not fluid overloaded there will be no haemodynamic compromise when unloading as Atherton showed [27].

## g)    Echocardiography

An immediate assessment by echocardiogram is pivotal due to the superior functional and diagnostic capability of this method [270–277, 287, 598].

# Chapter 2

## Acute heart failure syndromes

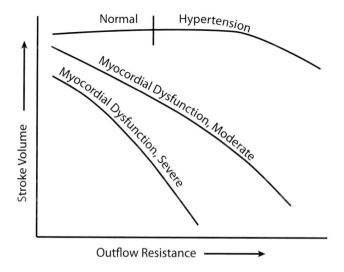

## 2.1    Definition

Poole-Wilson defines heart failure as, "a **clinical syndrome** due to ventricular dysfunction caused by an abnormality of the heart arising and accompanied by characteristic renal, neural and hormonal reactions" [1].

As yet no definition of heart failure is universally accepted, but Poole-Wilson describes all the relevant abnormalities caused by a primarily altered heart function.

The European Society of Cardiology (ESC) Task Force Group on **acute heart failure** defines it as, "the **rapid onset of symptoms and signs secondary to abnormal cardiac function.** It may occur with or without previous cardiac disease" [2].

## 2.2    Classification of acute heart failure syndromes (AHFS)

Acute heart failure may occur as an **acute *de novo* event** without previously known cardiac malfunction **or** as an **acute decompensation of chronic heart failure** [2].

The ESC Task Force Group has classified acute heart failure into six distinct pictures. This is based on the clinical conditions at presentation and the haemodynamic characteristics described by Forrester [3], Killipp [4] and more recently by Cotter [5], along with a report and explanation by Adams [6]:

- ESC- 1: **Acute Decompensated Heart Failure** (AD-HF)
  *De novo* or decompensated chronic HF.
  Signs and symptoms of acute HF are generally mild and do not fulfil criteria for cardiogenic shock (CS), pulmonary oedema or hypertensive crisis (HTN).
- ESC- 2: **Hypertensive Acute Heart Failure** (hypertensive AHF)
  Signs and symptoms of HF accompanied by high blood pressure (BP) and a chest radiograph compatible with acute pulmonary congestion but with relatively preserved ventricular function.

**Table 2.1** Haemodynamic profiles

|  | ESC-1 | ESC-2 | ESC-3 | ESC-4 | ESC-5 | ESC-6 |
|---|---|---|---|---|---|---|
| **Heart Rate** | = | ↑ | ↑ | ↑ | ↑ | ↓/↑ |
| **Systolic BP** | N/↑ | ↑/↑↑↑ | low N/↑ | N/↓−↓↓↓ | N/↓ | ↓/↓↓ |
| **Cardiac Index** [l/min/m²] | low N/↓ | N/↑/↓ | ↓ | < 1.8–2.2 −↓↓↓ | ↑/↑↑ | < 2.2 / ↓↓ |
| **PCWP** [mm Hg] | ↑, ≥ 12–16 | ↑, > 18 | ↑, > 16 | > 16 | N/↑ | < 12 |
| **Congestion** | +/++ | +/+++ | +++ | +/++ | −/+ | None |
| **Urine output** | −/+ | −/+ | + | low/None | +/− | low/None |
| **End Organ Hypoperfusion** | −/+ | −/+ | −/+ | ++/+++ | −/++ | −/+ |

- ESC- 3: **Pulmonary oedema**
  Symptoms and signs compatible with pulmonary oedema, normally accompanied by severe respiratory distress and $SaO_2$ usually <90% on room air prior to treatment with a chest X-ray showing pulmonary oedema.
- ESC- 4: **Cardiogenic Shock (CS)**
  The patient exhibits evidence of tissue hypoperfusion induced by HF after correction of pre-load. There is no clear definition of haemodynamic parameters, but CS is usually character-ised by reduced BP (systolic BP < 90 mm Hg or a drop of mean arterial pressure of > 30 mm Hg), and/or low urine output (< 0.5 ml/kg/h) with a pulse rate of > 60/min, with or without evidence of organ congestion.
  There is a continuum from low cardiac output syndrome to CS.
- ESC- 5: **High Output Failure**
  Characterised by high cardiac output, usually accompanied by tachycardia, warm peripher-ies, pulmonary congestion and sometimes a low BP as in septic shock. Main reasons for high output failure include septic shock, thyreotoxicosis, anaemia, Paget's disease and iatrogenic causes, e.g., catecholamine therapy.
- ESC-6: **Right Heart Failure (RV-HF)**
  Characterised as low output syndrome with ↑ jugular venous pressure, increased liver size, and hypotension.

## 2.3 Aetiology and epidemiology [2, 6–14]

The main causes of acute heart failure syndromes are:
- coronary (ischaemic) heart disease / ischemic cardiomyopathy,
- valvular heart disease,
- dilated cardiomyopathy,
- hypertension/hypertensive crisis and hypertrophic cardiomyopathy,
- acute arrhythmias,
- acute endocarditis,
- restrictive cardiomyopathy,
- acute pericarditis / cardiac tamponade,
- acute (peri) myocarditis,
- aortic dissection,
- **extracardiac diseases:**
  - broncho-pulmonary diseases, particularly those producing hypoxic states, e.g., acute ex-acerbation of COPD or severe pneumonia,
  - anaemia,
  - hyper/hypothyroidism, and other endocrine diseases,
  - fluid overload,
  - drug-induced heart failure,
  - metabolic/toxic reasons,
  - infectious diseases (particularly sepsis as high output heart failure),
  - neuromuscular diseases such as the myopathies,
  - trauma.

Coronary artery disease (CAD) is the **underlying cause of heart failure in the majority** of cases. Rudiger [12] conducted a European survey showing that CAD was the underlying disease in 62% of cases. Other studies have confirmed this showing CAD as the main aetiology of acute heart failure in 60–70% of cases [9–11, 13].

The vast majority of all patients admitted with acute heart failure (>60% [9] – 75% [6]) suffer from an **acute decompensation of chronic heart failure**, often decompensated due to systemic infection, pulmonary embolism, treatment with cardio-depressive drugs, reduction of the patient's cardio-specific medication or inappropriate physical stress [6, 9, 14]. Furthermore, up to 70% of all heart failure patients admitted suffer from arterial hypertension [6, 9, 15].

The main reason for acute HF in patients with 'preserved' systolic function, HFNEF, (EF > 50%) [16–18] is an acute increase in systolic blood pressure [19, 20], but new onset of atrial fibrillation (AF) is frequent as well [21].

Acute heart failure is the discharge diagnosis in about one million patients of all ages each year [22]. The in-hospital mortality is as high as 5% [23] and 33% will die within the first year following their first admission [24]. The five year mortality rate remains high, >50% [25].

The prognosis may be even worse as a recently published survey by Zinnad [13] revealed:

Contrary to other surveys, this French survey included not only patients suffering from acute heart failure admitted to general and cardiology wards but also severely ill patients requiring CCU or ITU admission. The number of patients with pulmonary oedema (82%) and cardio-genic shock (29%) was substantially higher than reported in previous studies [9, 10, 12]. The mortality in this study was as high as 27% at 4 weeks and 62.5% after one year.

## 2.4    Pathophysiology

### a)    The fundamental pathophysiological changes in acute heart failure syndromes

Acute decompensated chronic heart failure, pulmonary oedema, and hypertensive crisis (ESC-1, ESC-2 and ESC-3) are characterised by **progressive vasoconstriction** expressed by a markedly elevated peripheral vascular resistance and thus high vascular impedance during ventricular ejection [5, 26–29]. This exerts a **high end-systolic load on the myocardial wall** (high wall stress, see Chapter 1, paragraph 5) **which overlaps with impaired left ventricular function / functional reserve** [5, 26, 28, 29]. The consequence of this combination is a vicious circle of **afterload mismatch** with significantly reduced SV/CO and increased LVEDP [5, 30–34]. The elevated LVEDP affects the pulmonary capillaries and may precipitate pulmonary oedema [5, 32, 35].

Afterload ↑ and SV/CO ↓ and LVEDP ↑ [5, 30–35] (→ pulmonary oedema [31, 36])

Thus, the **fundamental pathophysiology in acute heart failure syndromes** is a **substantially elevated and inappropriate afterload** (afterload mismatch) **exerting a markedly elevated outflow resistance** / high impedance **on the LV during ventricular ejection** [26–28, 37].

SV reduction is either caused by the marked, **inappropriate** increase in afterload secondary to raised blood pressure and/or otherwise related to (peripheral) vasoconstriction [5, 37–39], with potentially an inflammatory process, or due to the compensatory activation of the sympathetic nervous system and the renin-angiotension-aldosterone system, leading to a significant and **inappropriate** elevation of systemic vascular resistance secondary to compromised systolic function (reduced contractility / impaired functional reserve) [26, 30, 40, 41].

In systolic HF (heart failure with reduced systolic function) with concomitant high afterload, the required increase in pressure generation by the LV can only be achieved by a disproportional increase in preload, thus by LV dilatation [42].

In heart failure with preserved systolic function (EF > 50%) [16–18], previously referred to as diastolic heart failure, (flash) pulmonary oedema is often caused by only a mild acute increase in blood pressure [35, 43–46] or even an undetectable volume expansion [47] **due to a deranged ventricular-arterial coupling** [35, 48, 49] as found in arterial stiffness [35, 50, 51], hence exerting an elevated systolic vascular load – afterload – on the LV. As a rule, arterial stiffness is accompanied by ventricular stiffening [35, 47, 49] or, if combined with pre-existing ventricular stiffness as in case of diastolic dysfunction [20, 35, 47, 52], the actual rise in blood pressure or volume stiffens the ventricle and leads to (further) ventricular stiffness [35, 47, 49, 53], inducing an acute rise in (the already elevated) systolic LV-load. This increase in systolic load prolongs the ventricular relaxation [46, 54] and compromises LV-filling [32]; the latter both induce a substantial increase in LVEDP [32, 46] which may lead to pulmonary oedema [31, 32, 35, 36] and, due to the marked increase in afterload, SV falls (afterload mismatch) [38].

The phenomenon of ventricular stiffening is seen in acute transient ischemia as well, and is another potential reason for acute pulmonary oedema independent of systolic LV function [55, 56]. For further details, see Chapter 5.

## b)    Pathophysiology and symptoms

The symptoms of heart failure are dominated by those related to congestion, a reflection of the elevated LVEDP [57]. Zinnad [13] found in his survey that 90% of all patients admitted with acute heart failure show signs of an elevated LVEDP.

**Elevated LVEDP** produces:
- ↑ oxygen-demand,
- compromised coronary perfusion giving an increased risk of global ischaemia, angina [30, 58] and subendothelial ischaemia [59],
- a strong neurohumeral response: ventricular stretch → further neurohumoral activation [60] → further ↑ LVEDP [30, 58, 61],
- **progressive mitral** (+/–tricuspid) **regurgitation** [62]. Significant **mitral regurgitation** (patients with symptoms at rest, thus NYHA IV) may fill as much as 50% of the total LV-SV [63].

A persistently high and therapy-resistant LVEDP is a predictor of increased risk for sudden decompensation and in-hospital death [30] and a therapeutic reduction of the LVEDP is correlated with improved outcome [30, 58, 64, 65]. An increased LVEDP is also the major determinate of consecutive right heart dysfunction [66].

It should be noted that acute severe left heart failure will not always by accompanied by high filling pressures (LVEDP). There are certainly some patients with normal or even low LVEDP's and no pulmonary oedema, although they do suffer from severe acute left heart failure [67–69] – this is so-called 'forward failure' by the ESC [2].

## 2.5    Data on clinical presentation and diagnosis

### a)       Presentation

- Proportion of clinical presentations of patients with heart failure syndromes [9, 13, 23]:
  - any dyspnoea           89%,
  - dyspnoea at rest        34%,
  - fatigue                32%,
  - rales on examination   68%,
  - peripheral oedema       66%,
  - X-ray congestion        75% (60–90% [13]).

Thus, symptoms are dominated by those related to congestion, reflecting the elevated LVEDP [57]; most commonly occurring are shortness of breath at rest or on minimal exertion, cough, orthopnoea, and paroxysmal nocturnal dyspnoea.

- Blood pressure on admission [6, 9, 23]:
  sBP   > 140 mm Hg       50% of all admissions,
  sBP   90–140 mm Hg     45% of all admissions,
  sBP   < 90 mm Hg        5% of all admissions.
- Dominant clinical conditions on admission to hospital in the Euro Heart Survey [9] (see ESC classification [2]):
  - 66% presented with the picture of **acute decompensated/exacerbated chronic HF,**
  - 17% showed **pulmonary oedema** as the dominating clinical condition,
  - 10% were admitted due to HF and **arterial hypertension,**
  - 4% with **cardiogenic shock,**
  - 3% were admitted due to an **acute right heart** problem.

As mentioned, the French survey [13] published in 2006 included the very sickest patients as well and recognised pulmonary oedema in 82% and cardiogenic shock in 29%.

### b)       Predictors of mortality

The **main predictors of high mortality were low systolic blood pressure (sBP) and elevated BUN at admission** [13, 70–72].

- **Blood pressure:**
  An analysis from the Optimize-Study by Gheorghiade [72] is shown in Table 2.2.
  - In the analysis of the ADHERE study data, a cut-off level of 125 mm Hg indicating a significantly worse prognosis was identified [70];
  - In the French survey [13], a sBP >120 mm Hg promised a better short term (four weeks) prognosis [13].

  Thus, a **systolic blood pressure (sBP) ≤ 120–125 mm Hg** should give cause for concern, and admission to a coronary care unit or high dependency unit should be considered.

Table 2.2 Optimize-study by Gheorghiade [72]

| sBP at admission | In-hospital mortality | 60–90 days mortality |
| --- | --- | --- |
| ≤ 119 mm Hg | 7.2% | 14.0% |
| 120–139 mm Hg | 3.6% | 8.4% |
| 140–161 mm Hg | 2.5% | 6.0% |
| ≥ 161 mm Hg | 1.7% | 5.4% |

Only 9.5% of all patients in the Optimize-HF study had an sBP < 104 mm Hg on admission.

- **Blood urea nitrogen:**
  BUN blood concentration > **37 mg/dl** [70] (urea > 13.2 mmol/l), > **43 mg/dl** [71] (urea > 15.35 mmol/l) is the other strong predictor of significantly increased mortality.

- **Other factors of concern but with less impact on the mortality are** [70]:
  - low serum sodium concentration,
  - elevated serum creatinine,
  - advanced age,
  - dyspnoea at rest,
  - chronic β-blocker use,
  - elevated troponin [73],
  - congestion at admission [74].

## c) Clinical haemodynamic profiles

A practical and helpful **clinical approach** to patients with **advanced acute heart failure** has been simplified by classifying the clinical scenario in to one of four haemodynamic profiles. Most patients can be classified during a two-minute bedside assessment [58, 75, 76] to a haemodynamic profile with corresponding treatment regimen [58]. The **main haemodynamic abnormalities are related to filling pressure and peripheral perfusion.** In the presence of **elevated filling pressures** the patient is said to be *'wet'*, in the absence *'dry'*; if the **perfusion of the peripheries** is adequate **'warm'**, if critically reduced **'cold'**. Note that the assessment concerning a 'cold' patient due to hypoperfusion should be made by assessing the legs and forearms rather than the feet and the hands [77].

Haemodynamic profiles are:
- **Profile 1: Warm and dry** → will not be seen in emergency admission unit. Requires therapy along standard chronic heart failure guidelines.
- **Profile 2: Warm and wet** (67% of all patients [78]) → initially nitroglycerin, but main step is to increase the dosage of their diuretic medication.
- **Profile 3: Wet and cold** (28% of all patients [78]) → warm the patient by using vasodilators (nitroglycerin or nitroprusside); when this is achieved, dry them with the aid of diuretics.
- **Profile 4: Cold and dry** → they are often surprisingly stable and are not usually seen in an emergency situation.

This clinical evaluation scheme and the treatment recommendations can be used and transferred to all clinical distinctions of AHFS.

**Clinical symptoms and signs of congestion (wet):** Jugular venous distension, peripheral oedema, hepatomegaly, crackles, rales, orthopnoea, paroxysmal nocturnal dyspnoea (due to systemic fluid retention) [2, 12].

**Clinical signs of hypoperfusion/shock (cold)** [58, 79, 80]: Altered level of consciousness (confused, quiet, apathetic), cold peripheries (forearms, lower leg), moist and clammy skin, mottled extremities, ↓ toe tip temperature, oliguria (renal dysfunction), ↓ MAP, hepatic dysfunction, low serum sodium.

The **cornerstones in making the diagnosis** are the patient's **history and clinical examination** [2, 81, 82].

Table 2.3 summarises the clinical haemodynamic profiles.

# d)     Echocardiography, X-ray, ECG and serum markers

Echocardiography, considered the "gold standard" for the detection of LV dysfunction [83], is an essential tool which should be performed rapidly to evaluate LV- function, structure, and any alterations to this; confirmation of the diagnosis is essential as well as identifying potentially reversible causes [2, 84].

The chest radiograph will aid diagnosis of congestion and/or pulmonary oedema [2, 82].

The electrocardiogram (ECG) will help to identify a precipitating ischemic event or the 'new' onset of atrial fibrillation inducing the AHFS [2, 82]. A normal ECG in a clinically suggested case of acute heart failure virtually rules out this diagnosis [85].

As the symptoms of acute heart failure may be non-specific and the physical findings sometimes not particularly sensitive [76, 86] the **Natriuretic Peptides**, ANP and BNP, may be helpful in the diagnosis, particularly in the emergency department [87–89].

The measurement of the serum level of natriuretic peptides is more or less established in the diagnosis and follow up of chronic heart failure [90, 91]. Their role is less clear in cases of acute heart failure, although an activation of various neurohumoral systems and, in particular, a rapid increase in ANP secondary to an acute elevation of the filling pressure is found in acute heart failure syndromes [92]. Acute stretch of the atria will release ANP [93], while BNP is predominantly liberated from the ventricles and is more strongly associated with chronic heart failure [94].

Nevertheless, Maisel [88] showed that BNP may be helpful in diagnosing acute heart failure in the emergency setting. In particular, the **excellent negative predictive value of BNP** can be used to exclude heart failure and potential cardiac failure from other underlying diseases [95] whilst the level of BNP also gives some information about the patient's prognosis [96–98], although this remains to be clarified [87].

**Troponin T and I** are highly sensitive and specific parameters allowing identification of myocardial injury and play a well-established key role in diagnosing acute coronary syndromes (ACS) [99] as well as in the risk stratification and management of patients suffering from ACS [100–103].

An elevation of cardiac troponin is found in about 40% of all patients with acute decompensated heart failure [104, 105], is associated with a low LV-EF [106, 107] and is said to predict a poor short term prognosis [106, 108].

Table 2.3 Clinical presentations of acute heart failure and cardiogenic shock

| WARM and DRY | WARM and WET ( > 50% of all patients) |
|---|---|
| **Clinical:** No specific HF symptoms; signs of severe infection/sepsis, tachycardia, hyperthyroid, etc; mild hypotension | **Clinical:** Symptoms dominated by the ↑ filling pressures causing shortness of breath – pulmonary congestion and/or acute and 'chronic' pulmonary oedema, peripheral oedema and ascites; $S_3$ is heard |
| **Haemodynamics:** sBP low n / n / ↑; CI n / ↑↑↑; PCWP n; hypoperfusion: None | **Haemodynamics:** sBP low n / ↑↑↑; CI (↓) / n / ↑; PCWP ↑ / ↑↑; hypoperfusion: None to mild; end organ hypoperfusion: (CNS) only in HTN |
| **Clinical scenarios most likely in this group:** ESC: ESC- 5, (ESC-1) | **Clinical scenarios most likely in this group:** ESC: ESC-1, ESC-2, ESC-3; (ESC-5) |
| **Key question:** Is the diagnosis of HF correct? | **Treatment:** Vasodilators and low dosages of diuretics |
| **Treatment:** Treat reason for high output: fluids; sepsis therapy etc. | |

| COLD and DRY | COLD and WET ( > 25% of all patients) |
|---|---|
| **Clinical:** Often stable, symptoms dominated by hypoperfusion such as altered level of consciousness, cold peripheries (forearms, lower leg), ↓ toe tip temperature, oliguria, ↓ MAP, (sometimes unappreciated congestion). | **Clinical:** Dominated by symptoms of hypoperfusion such as altered level of consciousness, cold peripheries (forearms, lower leg) with cold skin, moist and clammy, mottled extremities and ↓ toe tip temperature, oliguria, congestion/pulmonary oedema; ↓ MAP; $S_3$ heard; often caused by AMI |
| **Haemodynamics:** sBP ↓ / n; CI (low n) / ↓ / ↓↓↓; PCWP n / ↓; hypoperfusion: Mild to moderate | **Haemodynamics:** sBP ↓ / ↓↓↓; CI ↓ / ↓↓↓; PCWP ↑ / ↑↑↑; hypoperfusion: Mild to severe |
| **Clinical scenarios most likely in this group:** ESC: ESC-4a and 4b, ESC- 6 | **Clinical scenarios most likely in this group:** ESC: ESC- 4a and 4b (pre-shock* and manifest CS) |
| **Treatment:** Fluids, inotropes/vasopressors; see special RV failure treatment regime | * **Pre-shock criteria:** Hypoperfusion present but sBP > 90 mm Hg, crackles ≥ 50% of total lung area, pulmonary oedema, cold and sweaty patient, history of previous AMI. |
| | **Treatment:** Inotropes/vasopressors, IABP; Vasodilators only if SVR high |

You [109] has shown that troponin I is a strong predictor of all-cause mortality in patients with acute decompensated heart failure. The study shows an independent 'dose'-response relationship between cardiac troponins and mortality in AHFS-patients. Thus, an association between elevated cardiac troponins and poor outcome in acute heart failure seems to be established.

## e)      The CPI–SVRI relation

The diagnosis of acute heart failure may still be difficult due to non-specific symptoms and insensitive physical findings [76, 86]. As such, the haemodynamic assessment of patients with signs of acute failure is still regarded as the most accurate and sensitive method with which to establish the exact diagnosis with the highest accuracy [110]. Cotter [5] established proof that by combining SVRI and CPI using a special algorithm, the exact diagnosis can be achieved in up to 95% of patients. (Note that, CPI and SVRI may be achieved non-invasively with reasonable accuracy [111]) (see Figure 1.13).

## 2.6      Therapy [2, 76, 79, 112–127]

## a)      Therapeutic principles and goals

The **immediate** goals of managing an emergent case are [30, 58, 76]:
- rapid stabilisation,
- symptom relief,
- reversal of the haemodynamic abnormalities, in particular:
    - reduction of the elevated LVEDP (determines the outcome [30, 58, 64]),
    - significant reduction of the increased afterload (main underlying pathophysiology) [5, 26, 28],
    - ↑ of the SV/CO.

Remember:
- afterload ↓ → **LVEDP** ↓ [128];
  when afterload ↓ → LVEDP ↓ [119, 129] → diastolic wall stress ↓ → $O_2$-requirement ↓ [38, 130] → **LVEDD** ↓ [119, 129, 130],
- afterload ↓ → **SV/CO** ↑ [28].
The failing heart is exquisitely sensitive to afterload [29, 131] and so a reduction in the LV outflow impedance (afterload) impeding the ejection by pharmacological vasodilatation will improve the LV ejection, is substantially validated and is the rational therapeutic approach of choice in acute left heart failure [132, 133].

There is growing evidence that the best therapeutic approach is:
**Early intravenous vasodilators** (GTN, nesiritide, nitroprusside) and **low dose** diuretics [30, 134–136].
Vasodilators exert a direct effect on the elevated filling pressures and the increased afterload

providing a 'physiological' therapeutic approach [30, 135]. Vasodilators promote the rapid nor-malisation of the altered haemodynamics and there is evidence that intravenous administration of vasodilators in the emergency department reduces [30, 65, 137]:
- **in-hospital mortality,**
- the length of hospital stay,
- the necessity for invasive diagnostic and therapeutic procedures.

A **reduction in afterload** will, as a rule, lead to a proper increase in flow (SV/CO), prevent-ing the development of hypotension, thus the MAP will be maintained or may increase but will not fall [27, 138, 139]. Concerns that the reduction of a severely elevated filling pressure and afterload could reduce the SV (and thus CO and BP) are completely unwarranted:
In daily clinical practice when the peripheral resistance (afterload) is lowered by administra-tion of vasodilating agents, the LV wall stress (end-diastolic and end-systolic) will be reduced [119, 129]. Simultaneously the SV will increase due to the reduction in afterload [28, 140] with an increase in forward flow [138, 141–143]. Furthermore, particularly in severe dilated heart failure, the reduction in LV outflow resistance and filling pressures leads to a concomi-tant substantial decrease in MR causing a marked increase in SV/CO [128, 130, 141, 142–145].
If, with this approach, the blood pressure **cannot be maintained** and there is no increase in SV/CO **one of the following circumstances** should be considered and treated:
- **severe mitral regurgitation** [62, 63, 130, 146, 147],
- inappropriate filling volume (LVEDV) [130, 144, 148],
- matching of the ventriculo-arterial coupling [149, 150] (see Chapter 1, paragraph 9),
- relatively low intravascular volume (relative hypovolaemia) [112, 151] – seldom.

A marked reduction in afterload and LVEDP will, as mentioned, significantly increase the LV-forward output [141–143] and will substantially reduce the regurgitant orifice and the grade of MR [63, 152, 153]. The use of nitroprusside infusion or diuretics has shown to decrease the grade of MR by up to 50% [130, 152].

Several recently published large studies [12, 13, 70, 72] have all found that a sBP < 120 mm Hg is a strong indicator of poor (short term) outcome. Hypotension impairs autoregulation [154, 155] and, if persistent, will aggravate any myocardial perfusion deficit [156] and play a part in a vicious cycle leading to a more and more severely ischaemic myocardium [157, 158], worsening the situation. Therefore caution is recommended in initiating vasodilator therapy or drugs with vasodilative effects (i.e. Dobutamine, Levosimendan) if sBP < 120 mm Hg.
Nevertheless, as long as there is clear evidence of elevated peripheral resistance and LVEDP, low dosages under close and continuous monitoring seem to be appropriate because a reduction of afterload is the pathophysiological approach of choice and recent publications and guidelines recommend the use of vasodilators in clinically stable patients even with sBP of 95 mm Hg [159–161] and the ESC accepts a sBP as low as 85 mm Hg [2, 122].
Nitroglycerin in low doses (< 0.5 μg/kg/min) is known not to decrease peripheral blood pres-sure or to compromise peripheral perfusion but it reduces the aortic (central) blood pressure and thus the systolic load directly faced by the ventricle [162, 163].
[It must be remembered that a sBP < **90 mm Hg**, in conjunction with a typical underlying condition and appropriate clinical signs of hypoperfusion is a criterion of cardiogenic **shock**

[79, 80, 164, 165] and therefore in the summary diagram you will find 90 mm Hg as a cut off for hypotension.]

Additional information for a logical therapeutic approach can be extracted from the study by Cotter on 'The role of cardiac power index and systemic vascular resistance in the pathophysiology and diagnosis of patients with acute congestive heart failure' [5]. He not only confirmed the well established pathophysiology of acute heart failure syndromes – showing the validity and quality of his results – but showed how the relation between the actual pump function (expressed by CPI) and the corresponding afterload (expressed by the size of the peripheral resistance) can and should be used in the daily therapeutic decision process. In his diagram he plotted the paired parameters (CPI – SVRI) as a two-dimensional graph. This can be used for diagnostic purpose (see Figure 1.13) but also for the choice of appropriate therapy as well:

The SVRI in relation to CPI (cardiac function) is inappropriately high (afterload mismatch) in clinical situations such as pulmonary oedema or hypertensive crisis as well as in the majority of acutely exacerbated chronic heart failure patients (SVRI roughly 3000 with normal values of 1970–2390 dynes/sec/cm$^{-5}$ [166–168]). If the SVRI is (very) high in relation to the cardiac function parameter, a vasodilator will be the treatment of choice and this is even the case with a relatively low blood pressure [5].

In the presence of cardiogenic shock the SVRI is inappropriately low, not compensating for the markedly reduced cardiac function (expressed by a low CPI) [26, 30, 40, 41]. This leads to a critically low blood pressure and significant hypoperfusion, hence vasopressors may be necessary [5, 116, 117, 152, 169]. Hypotension in this situation reflects failure of the sympathetic nervous system to compensate circulatory shock, whilst normotension does not ensure haemodynamic stability [170].

The different therapeutic recommendations given in this book are based on a number of different relationships. The relationship between cardiac function/performance and vascular resistance/afterload is crucial; the heart in a failing state is exquisitely sensitive to afterload [29, 131–133], and the LV afterload is the decisive determinant of cardiac performance in heart failure [28, 29, 171]. In cardiogenic shock or pre-shock the compensatory vasoconstriction is, in most patients, inappropriate in relation to the loss of performance [5, 172–174] (see Chapter 3) and, of course, there is a necessity to avoid life-threatening deterioration due to (further) myocardial ischemia with (further) depression of contractility secondary to low systemic blood pressure and reduced coronary perfusion pressure [156–158]. In such cases the use of vasopressor and inotropic medications may be unavoidable, but it must be remembered that the use of inotropes in patients with relatively preserved LV-function (EF > 40%) has shown a higher mortality [120, 126, 136, 175–177].

Ejection fraction is the most widely used parameter of LV systolic function [178, 179], and so we shall also use EF (and CPI). An EF of > 40% is generally accepted as representing relatively preserved systolic LV function [23, 136, 180–186].

A similarly accepted standard benchmark for a sufficient CPI has not yet been adopted. Based on the diagram provided by Cotter [5], current publications [187] and extrapolating the fact that a CPO ≤ 0.53 [110] clearly indicates high risk patients, we suggest that a **CPI of > 0.3** in case of reduced, normal or mildly/moderately increased SVRI (up to around 3000) seems to be the lowest limit acceptable. With a higher SVRI, lower CPIs may be appropriate, with the diagram by Cotter [5] depicting a CPI of 0.2 being above the limit indicating shock when the SVRI is equal or above 9000 dynes/sec/cm$^{-5}$.

For practical purposes, a copy of the diagram by Cotter may be of value to carry in your pocket when on call.

# b)    Treatment of underlying disease [112–117]:

- primary angioplasty or thrombolysis of acute ST-elevation myocardial infarction,
- percutaneous coronary intervention (PCI) in patients suffering from refractory myocardial ischaemia,
- antibiotic treatment for patients with endocarditis,
- pericardiocentesis in order to relieve cardiac tamponade caused by trauma, acute pericarditis, malignancy or other cause,
- treatment of acute arrhythmias (i.e. pacemaker, anti arrhythmic drugs, acute ablation),
- urgent surgical intervention on complications of myocardial infarction or aortic dissection,
- antibiotic treatment for systemic infectious diseases with heart failure as a complication.

# c)    Essential measures

The patient should be assessed according to the ABC (airway, breathing, circulation) method of resuscitation, which tends to be standard but with emphasis on particular areas:
- The patient should sit upright;
- If peripheral $O_2$-saturation is < 90% [112, 188], administer oxygen, 2.5 to 10 L to achieve a normal saturation of 95 to 98% (Class I recommendation, evidence level C [2]). A saturation of <90% is an important sign that the patient most probably has pulmonary oedema [159] – these patients should be classified as 'wet' [75, 76].
  (**NB**. Hyperoxygenation can be associated with reduced coronary blood flow, increased systemic resistance, reduced cardiac output and shows a trend to higher mortality [189, 190].
- Morphine sulphate: 1 to 3 mg IV, may be repeated several times (Class II b recommendation, Evidence level B [2]).

## i)    Vasodilators

*Nitroglycerin (GTN)*
This is indicated as **first line therapy** [120, 134, 135, 191, 192] in all patients as long as the systolic BP > 95–100 [159, 160] – some authors require a systolic pressure > 85 mm Hg [2, 122, 193], MAP > 60–70 mm Hg [122, 159].

Dosage: 20 µg/min up to 200 µg/min. (Class I recommendation, evidence level A [117, 171] or B [2]), Leier [161] states that a systolic BP > 95 mm Hg is high enough to initiate a GTN infusion of 0.3–0.5 µg/kg/min. GTN-resistance can be remedied by increasing doses [194]. In case of phosphodiesterase 5-inhibitor treatment, GTN is contraindicated [195].

Note that even very low doses (<0.5 µg/kg/min) of GTN will decrease the LV wall stress (end-diastolic and end-systolic) with reduction of the aortic (central) blood pressure (direct afterload faced by the ventricle), but without a detectable drop of pressure or perfusion in the periphery (tissue perfusion) – a very welcome and desirable effect [162, 163].

*Nitroglycerin* has clear advantages *compared to diuretics* as a first line drug. It is not only more effective than diuretics in controlling severe pulmonary oedema [159] but has a more balanced haemodynamic profile [30, 135] with faster reduction in wall stress and LVEDP without reducing the CO [196]. GTN gives beneficial results without significant side effects [197], whilst diuretics may produce complications due to reduction of glomerular filtration rate (GFR) [198] and a further activation of the neurohumoral system [128, 191, 199] with amplification of vasoconstriction and thus may induce a (further) decrease in SV [135]. High dosages of loop diuretics (i.e. furosemide) may even lead to AMI and death; their use has, in some studies, shown an increased in-hospital and overall mortality rate [135, 159, 191, 192].

Always keep in mind that not all patients with pulmonary oedema are fluid overloaded [200, 201] and as such have no indication for diuretics.

An induction of (relative) hypovolaemia or a deterioration of a persistent (relative) hypovolaemia secondary to use of diuretics [200, 201] can cause harm, with a negative effect on the outcome [136, 191, 202, 203].

### Nitroprusside

Nitroprusside is a potent venous and arterial vasodilator [204] and is extremely effective in reducing the afterload as well as reducing the pre-load, and thus lowering end-systolic and end-diastolic wall stress [142]. It decreases the neurohumoral activation markedly (an important underlying pathological mechanism) [205]. In patients where the systolic BP exceeds 120 mm Hg, and particularly in hypertensive crises, the use of nitroprusside should be seriously considered [40], and some authors recommend it [2, 204]. A further important indication is severe mitral regurgitation [63, 152, 153].

Dosage 0.3 µg/kg/min to 5.0 µg/kg/min. (Class I recommendation, evidence level C [2] or A [117, 171]).

Nitroprusside has substantial dose dependent arterial dilating effects which, in the case of fixed arterial narrowing, may cause a significant reduction in blood flow distal to the stenotic area, a so-called 'steal-phenomenon' [204]. Hence, it may cause a regional decrease in coronary flow [206–208] in patients with CAD. In acute myocardial infarction, nitroprusside should not be used because ischaemia may be worsened, inducing or exacerbating left sided heart failure [209].

### Nesiritide

A novel approach in the treatment of acute left heart failure is **nesiritide.** It is chemically identical to human BNP acting via cGMP to produce a balanced (arterio-venous) vasodilatation, i.e. a pre- and afterload/wall stress (end-diastolic and end-systolic) reduction [210, 211]. There is an increase in SV/CO without direct inotropic effect [189, 212], enhanced sodium excretion and suppression of the renin-angiotensin-aldosterone axis as well as of the sympathetic nervous system [2, 194, 197, 212, 213]. A beneficial effect on renal function [214] and an enhanced diuresis has been demonstrated [197, 212].

Dosage: Initial 2 µg/kg bolus, followed by 0.01 µg/kg/min infusion [197, 215]

Nesiritide is thought to be safe; its use does not require ICU admission or invasive monitoring and it is associated with a low incidence of tachycardia and arrhythmias [137, 212, 216, 217]. The initial studies using nesiritide as a first line drug in acute heart failure treatment were very encouraging [120, 197, 213, 218] and, in Japan, it is the preferred drug in acute heart failure therapy [219]. Compared to the classical inotropic drugs, particularly to dobutamine, nesiritide shows fewer arrhythmias and a better outcome [120, 218, 216, 217].

In comparison to nitroglycerin the haemodynamic improvements (reduction of LVEDP and thus pulmonary hypertension) [194,197] of nesiritide are even more intensive and the relief of the patients' dyspnoea is more rapid [197, 213]. There are even fewer side effects, although this did not translate into better mortality outcomes [120, 197]. Unfortunately, a recently published meta-analysis by Sakner-Bernstein described a trend to a higher mortality in the group treated with nesiritide compared to standard therapy (GTN and diuretics) [220].

Nesiritide may be recommended as therapy in cases complicated by renal failure and for patients with signs of congestion but with adequate perfusion [214]. Thus, in patients without shock, patients should be 'warm'.

### ii)        Diuretics and continuous renal replacement therapy (CRRT)
Diuretics directly reduce excess levels of extracellular fluid [30]. They **indirectly** exert haemodynamic effects and reduce the LVEDP by venodilation [221], hence promoting the relief of symptoms caused by congestion [30, 134]. Loop diuretics given IV commence their diuretic effect after approximately 30 minutes with the venodilating effects commencing 15 minutes after administration and with actions lasting up to two hours [222]. Diuretics are **indicated** in patients with acute left heart failure who show **symptoms secondary to fluid retention / fluid overload** [2, 134–136].

Diuretics are not a first line drug and a diuretic based approach has significant limitations, not least due to the aforementioned adverse outcome [2, 134, 135, 191, 192, 223]. They should be added in low dosage in fluid overloaded patients after vasodilator therapy has been initiated [30, 134–136].

Dosage: Start with 20 to 40 mg IV [134, 123, 193], 80 mg if serum creatinine > 200 µmol/l [118]. (Class I recommendation, evidence level A [117, 171], evidence level B by the ESC [2]).

Avoid higher dose boluses (> 1 mg/kg) which may induce reflex vasoconstriction [224] and worsen the vascular resistance.

A Cochrane analysis by Salvador [225] established that a continuous infusion of loop diuretics provides a larger diuresis and greater safety than intermittent bolus doses. In patients resistant to therapy a poorer prognosis is seen [226]. In this scenario further options include using a furosemide infusion [227], bumetanide [228] or a combination of furosemide and metolazone [229, 230].

Torasemide (atypical loop diuretic agent [207]) has shown a better functional improvement, a lower incidence of hypokalaemia and a lower mortality [207] when compared with furosemide and other loop diuretics [231]. It produces a lower transcardiac aldosterone gradient due to mineralocorticoid receptor blocking effects [232].

**Continuous renal replacement therapy** (continuous ultrafiltration – UF) should be considered at an **early** point in patients with acute severe heart failure who are fluid overloaded, show an inadequate response to diuretic therapy, are oligo-anuric [122, 233, 234] and/or have deteriorating renal failure as described by Mehta [191] and others [233, 235]. The **Unload Trial** (Ultrafiltration vs Diuretics for Patients Hospitalised for Acute Decompensated Chronic Heart Failure) [235] is the first study showing the superiority in clinical outcomes of the ultrafiltration group compared to the diuretic group. Furthermore, very progressively, **peripheral venous access** and new, small sized ultrafiltration equipment was used. Two further small trials confirmed these results, stating that using peripheral ultrafiltration more fluid was removed and renal function was no further compromised compared with diuretic therapy [236, 237]. Thus, a broader application of this safe technique seems to be appropriate [238].

The deterioration of renal function in AHFS is multifactorial, aside from acute changes in central haemodynamics [62, 239–241] and the neuroendocrine activation [60, 77] there are multiple other processes involved that compromise renal function, including the so-called cardio-renal link [62, 239, overview by 242]. Fluid regulation, removal of mediators (especially of cardiac depressant factors [243]) and resetting of homeostasis (electrolytes, acid-base balance) are the three main beneficial aspects of haemofiltration [244]. With UF you avoid the negative effects of diuretic drugs [120, 191, 245].

It should be stressed that continuous UF has in fluid overloaded patients, if any at all, a **minimal effect on MAP** [233, 235, 244, 246].

### iii)      Inotropic drugs and vasopressor therapy

Inotropic drugs are conventionally used to increase CO (SV) and improve peripheral and organ perfusion [81, 134] in cases of low output, hypoperfusion and in life threatening situations [5, 117, 152, 190].

In recent years the use of inotropic drugs has been overshadowed by growing, clear evidence of adverse clinical outcome and increased mortality [115, 120, 175, 193, 217, 218], particularly in patients with reasonably [2] preserved left ventricular function (LV-EF > 40%) [120, 126, 136, 175–177]. Conners [247] and Sandham [248] found a significantly increased mortality when clinically stable patients were treated with conventional inotropic agents due to numerically low cardiac output. The ADHERE register [120] revealed that the use of dobutamine or milrinone compared to GTN led to a significantly higher mortality in the treatment of AHFS [120, 249].

The potential danger of catecholamines is due to their effect of increasing the myocardial oxygen requirement and overloading the myocytes with calcium [48].

Only patients who absolutely require inotropic support due to (potential) hypoperfusion secondary to low output as the result of a severely reduced contractility and who are resistant to other treatment attempts should be treated by such agents [70, 136, 250].

The ESC [2] recommends inotropic agents if the disease (AHFS) has deteriorated to a life threatening setting where the situation becomes critically dependent on the haemodynamics: 'Inotropic agents are indicated in the presence of peripheral hypoperfusion with or without congestion or pulmonary oedema refractory to vasodilators and diuretics at optimal dosages'.

When considering inotropic drugs the use of **intra-aortic balloon counterpulsation (IABP)** should also be considered [2, 117, 251]; the IABP has become a standard component in the treatment of patients suffering from cardiogenic shock or severe left heart failure [2, 117, 252–254].

*Inotropic agents*

**Dobutamine** can be considered in hypotension due to markedly reduced contractility. This should be persistent despite optimised pre-and afterload, with the afterload in the normal/mild to moderately elevated range and with a systolic BP as low as ≥ 70 mm Hg, if there are no (further) clinical signs of shock to be found [151]. Most authors prefer a higher blood pressure limit of 80–85 mm Hg as a prerequisite to commencing dobutamine [2, 117, 255–257]. As long as the patient is euvolaemic, a blood pressure drop due to the peripheral vasodilatory effects of dobutamine is rare because the peripheral vasodilation will generally be compensated for by the increase in CI/SV (forward flow) [141–143, 258].

Dobutamine has positive inotropic and chronotropic effects [259, 260]. It decreases the sympathetic tone producing reduced peripheral resistance [261] (↓ wall stress, i.e. ↓ afterload) without a significant drop in MAP due to compensatory ↑ SV / ↑ CI [2]. Dobutamine is associated with an increased risk of arrhythmia [216, 223] and it may worsen the splanchnic tissue perfusion [262]. Although it usually decreases pulmonary wedge pressure (PCWP) there are patients in whom PCWP remains unchanged or even increases [116]. Higher dosages of dobutamine will cause vasoconstriction [206].

Dosage: 2 to 20 µg/kg/min, usually initiated at 2–3 µg/kg/min [2].

After 24 to 48 hours of use patients develop tolerance with partial loss of haemodynamic effects [116].

**Dopamine** is recommended if the patient has developed cardiogenic shock, if the sBP is < 70 mm Hg [190, 263] or in unstable patients with a sBP between ≥ 70 and 80 mm Hg [117, 264–266]. The combination of dobutamine and dopamine is validated as being the first choice in the treatment of cardiogenic shock [116, 117, 255]. There is clear evidence that the combination of dopamine and dobutamine improves the haemodynamic situation [267].

Dopamine stimulates dose related dopamine-receptors (≤ 2–3 µg/kg/min), β-receptors (> 2 µg/kg/min) causing a positive inotropic and chronotropic effect, and α-receptors (> 5 µg/kg/min) causing vasoconstriction [2, 268, 269].

However, dopamine has many adverse effects including the induction of lethal arrhythmias [270], cardiomyocyte calcium overload precipitating apoptosis [270], increase in afterload, increase in pulmonary resistance [175], deterioration in the oxygenation of the mucosa (which is at high risk of hypoxia in such situations) and of the intestine [271], intestinal motility disturbances [271] and restriction of the vascular supply to the thyroid and myocardium [272] due to its vasoconstrictive effects – all of which potentially increase mortality [190, 193, 219, 273].

**Noradrenaline** shows fewer side effects [272, 274, 275] compared to dopamine and should be the **preferred vasopressor** when substantial vasoconstrictive effects are rapidly needed [169, 274, 276–280] i.e. patients who are either clinically or haemodynamically unstable and in life-threatening situations with severe hypotension and/or hypoperfusion [116, 117, 121, 152, 169].

Critical hypotension itself will further compromise the myocardial perfusion and will markedly increase the LVEDP (vicious cycle). This may precipitate a life-threatening situation [117, 152, 274]. The ESC [2] recommends vasopressor therapy in AHFS when initial therapy including inotropic agent(s) and fluid challenge has (have) failed to restore arterial and end organ perfusion despite improvement in cardiac output.

Noradrenaline is certainly more effective than dopamine in reversing systemic hypotension [274, 278, 280]. It has been found to improve and secure organ and tissue perfusion. Blood supply to the kidneys [281–283] and the heart muscle [281, 284]; perfusion of the stomach and the whole gut [285, 286] seems to be less (or even not) compromised when reasonable doses of NA are used in preference to dopamine.

With increased MAP, autoregulation of the kidneys [282] and the heart (coronary perfusion) [281, 284] will be re-established.

If necessary, a combination of noradrenaline and dobutamine will improve the haemodynamic situation significantly and should, based on current evidence, be preferred to the combination of dopamine plus dobutamine [2, 117, 127, 169, 287, 288]. The use of dopamine or adrenaline is also associated with a **significantly higher mortality rate compared to noradrenaline and dobutamine** [289].

**Phosphodiesterase inhibitors** are indicated in cases of peripheral hypoperfusion with or without congestion, refractory to diuretics and vasodilators at optimal dose, and with preserved systemic blood pressure (sBP > 80–85 mm Hg) [2, 117, 255–257]. They show positive inotropic, lusiotropic as well as vasodilatory effects with improvement of SV/CO and reduction of the systemic (afterload) and pulmonary resistance [117, 290]. Due to their site of action (via intracellular inhibition of type III phosphodiesterase thus increasing cardiac cAMP concentration, the second messenger used for intracellular signal transduction [291, 292]) they may be administered even if the patient is on β- blockers [293, 294]. Unfortunately, there is growing evidence that phosphodiesterase-inhibitors increase mortality and complications when compared with other treatment regimes (vasodilators, diuretics, levosimendan) [120, 175, 295–297].

Dosage of milrinone: 25 μg/kg bolus over 10 to 20 min., followed by an infusion of 0.375 to 0.75 μg/kg/min [2].

**Levosimendan** is a newly developed agent acting as a calcium-sensitiser which may become the drug of choice in the treatment of hypoperfusion due to 'symptomatic low cardiac output and left heart failure secondary to cardiac systolic dysfunction' [2].

Myocardial contractility is ultimately determined by the effects of calcium on the actin-myosin complex. Calcium-sensitisers, 'sensitise' the actin-myosin complex to the effect of calcium [298].

Levosimendan will increase the contractility of the heart by increasing the stability of the calcium-troponin-complex in the cardiac myocyte without increasing the intracellular ionized calcium concentration (as catecholamines and phosphodiesterase inhibitors do) [299, 300]. Levosimendan has vasodilatory effects with peripheral vasodilation, producing a reduction in afterload and of end-systolic wall stress which is beneficial in terms of the underlying pathophysiology [301]. Levosimendan also exerts positive effects on the diastolic function, it improves the diastolic components [302, 303].

Therefore, in comparison to catecholamines and phosphodiesterase-inhibitors, levosimendan does not impair diastolic relaxation, avoiding an increase in myocardial stiffness and consecutively impaired LV compliance with the effect of increasing LVEDP [304–306].

Recent studies [295, 307–310] underline the favourable and beneficial effects of levosi-

Table 2.4  Modified from ESC Guidelines on acute heart failure [2] and others [115, 116, 120–127]

**WARM and DRY**

Patient normally compensated.
In high output cardiac failure treat the underlying disease.

**WARM and WET**

| sBP ≥ 90(95)–120 mm Hg | | sBP > 120–160 | sBP > 160 | Vasodilators |
|---|---|---|---|---|
| EF ≤ 0.4 / CPI ≤ 0.3 +/or SVR ↓/n/(↑)  →  LEV(DOB) | EF > 0.4 / CPI > 0.3 + SVR ↑/↑↑  →  gtn or NES | GTN or NES (or Niprus) | Niprus or GTN | GTN (low dose: gtn) |
| + diuretics after stabilisation if appropriate | | + diuretics | + diuretics | Nitroprusside (Niprus) |
| | | | | Nesiritide (NES) |
| | | | | Diuretics (always low dose, max. 40 mg, as initial dose) or Haemofiltration |

**COLD and DRY**

Haemodynamic monitoring essential

Fluids, if evidence of hypovolemia and positive response to fluids by dynamic fluid responsiveness test is confirmed as well as EVLWI < 10; furthermore, if no signs for DVI and isolated/predominating RV-failure.

| sBP ≥ 90(95)–100 | | sBP < 90–70 | sBP < 70 |
|---|---|---|---|
| SVR ↑-↑↑ and EF > 0.4 / CPI > 0.3 | EF ≤ 0.4 / CPI ≤ 0.3 | CS-situation see Chapters 3/4 | CS-situation see Chapters 3/4 |
| gtn or NES if BP ↓, stop gtn/NES, consider LEV/DOB ± NA | LEV/DOB stop LEV/DOB, if BP↓ or add NA | | |

**COLD and WET**

Haemodynamic monitoring essential

Patient stable, but potentially in pre-shock.

| sBP < 90 | | sBP ≥ 90 | |
|---|---|---|---|
| Cardiogenic shock / pre-shock situation see Chapter 3 | SVR n/↓ and/or EF ≤ 0.4 / CPI ≤ 0.3 | SVR ↑-↑↑ but EF ≤ 0.4 / CPI ≤ 0.3 | SVR n/↑-↑↑ and EF > 0.4 / CPI > 0.3 |
| | LEV or DOB add NA if BP↓ | LEV or DOB if BP↓ stop LEV/DOB (or add NA) | NES or gtn if BP↓ consider LEV or DOB and/or stop NES/gtn |

Inotropic Agents: Dobutamine (DOB), Levosimendan(LEV) [127, 288, 307–310] and Vasopressor Noradrenaline (NA), mechanical support IABP [252–254, 344, 345].

mendan in the treatment of acute left heart failure syndromes, particularly in patients with post-myocardial infarction left heart failure and acute decompensated chronic heart failure. The 'CASINO'-study showed that patients who were treated by levosimendan experienced a significantly lower mortality rate compared to those treated with dobutamine, milrinone or to the placebo-group [311].

Results from the REVIVE [312] and SURVIVE I & II [313] studies – although not as convincing as expected – do not contradict the fact that the mortality rates of levosimendan are significantly lower than when using dobutamine or phosphodiesterase-inhibitors, if the correct patient and indication is taken into consideration: **Patients with acutely exacerbated chronic heart failure** (the vast majority of patients) in need of inotropic support [312–314], **patients with acute heart failure who are on β-blockers** [312–314] and **acute heart failure complicating AMI** [309, 314]. Furthermore, levosimendan is shown to be applicable in combination with noradrenaline in case of cardiogenic shock [288, 315–317]. So, on current evidence, levosimendan is validated at evidence level **B** [2], Class IIa recommendation [2] whilst all other inotropic agents are rated level C.

Most authors recommend an sBP of at least 85 mm Hg in otherwise stable patients (in particular if the peripheral vascular resistance is normal or low) as a necessary prerequisite to commencing levosimendan in order to avoid a further BP drop due to its vasodilative abilities [2, 318, 319]. The potential for a blood pressure drop can be minimised by avoiding hypovolaemia prior to starting the infusion of levosimendan [316].

Dosage [318]: Loading dose 12 μg/kg–24 μg/kg administered over 10 min followed by a continuous infusion of 0.05 to 0.1 μg/kg/min, up titrated to max. 0.2 μg/kg/min for 6 to 24 hours. If there are concerns of inducing a blood pressure drop, levosimendan may be initiated without a loading dose.

### iv)      Arrhythmias and heart failure

There is an increased incidence of ventricular [320] and supraventricular arrhythmias, particularly atrial fibrillation and flutter [321] in chronic congestive heart failure. Ventricular arrhythmias are associated with an elevated risk of sudden death and non-arrhythmic death [322, 323]. The new onset of an arrhythmia during the exacerbation of chronic heart failure characterises a high-risk patient group with increased morbidity and mortality in the short and long-term [324]. While the severity of heart failure does not predict the likelihood of the development of new arrhythmias, there is a strong relation between the use of inotropic drugs and the onset of new arrhythmias [324].

40% of all new arrhythmias are atrial fibrillation (AF) [324]. New onset of AF is associated with a significant clinical and haemodynamic deterioration [325], increased risk of death [326, 327] and conversion to sinus rhythm lowers the mortality rate [327]. Amiodarone is shown to be beneficial because of its effectiveness and only mild negative inotropic side effects in heart failure patients with arrhythmias [328–331].

### v)      Continuous positive airway pressure (CPAP) and non-invasive (positive pressure) ventilatory support (NIPPV)

CPAP is indicated in acute heart failure patients who, despite oxygen delivered via face mask and drug therapy, are still de-saturated ($SaO_2$ < 90%) [2] and where the patient is exhausted from the high respiratory workload required due to pulmonary congestion [332–334]. By decreasing the **left-ventricular afterload** and the respiratory work, CPAP improves oxygenation, decreases symptoms and significantly reduces the need for endotracheal intubation and mechanical ventilation [335–339]. A statistically significant reduction of mortality has not been shown as yet, probably due to the small populations studied. However, a systematic review has found a trend towards decreased in-hospital mortality [334, 340]. CPAP: Class II a recommendation, evidence level A of the ESC [2].

NIPPV is more helpful in hypercapnic pulmonary oedema, where there is failure of respiratory musculature as well. A recent study found NIPPV was at least as effective as CPAP, but the effect of unloading the respiratory muscles led neither to a lower rate of endotracheal intubation nor to a shortened recovery time [341].

#### vi)      Anticoagulation

Prophylactic anticoagulation with low molecular weight heparin (LMWH) or unfractionated heparin is strongly recommended (although substantial evidence is still lacking) in order to prevent thrombo-embolic complications [122, 252, 342]. Dosage: 40 mg enoxaparin (or equivalent) s. c. or 5000 Units unfractionated Heparin s. c. × 3 daily [343].

## 2.7      Valvular heart diseases presenting as heart failure [overview 346, 347]

Acute heart failure due to valvular disease is found in 4% [348] to 24% [12] of all patients admitted with the clinical picture of an AHFS.

## a)      Mitral regurgitation

Acute MR is a serious emergency situation, as flash pulmonary oedema may occur [347]. The main causes of acute MR are rupture or insufficiency of a papillary muscle (mostly posterior) due to acute myocardial infarction (AMI) or rupture of the chordae tendinae as a complication of AMI, endocarditis, chest trauma and myxomatous degeneration of the valve [349].

Main pathophysiology:
Acute pressure increase in the **non-adapted LA** due to regurgitation leads to an increased pressure in the pulmonary circulation and thus pulmonary congestion/oedema [36, 350].

The left ventricular ejection is bidirectional [146, 351], the regurgitation area is often dynamic and depends on the dimension of the LV [146]. The increased diastolic volume induces, via the Frank-Starling mechanism, an increase in SV, but due to the bidirectional ejection the effective SV (forward output) will be reduced [347].

In case of chronic MR, where the heart and in particular the LA are adapted, the acute decompensation is most often due to muscle failure, triggered by acute arterial hypertension, acute myocardial ischaemia and arrhythmias such as the new onset of uncontrolled AF [347].

Special therapeutic aspects:
• In **acute MR nitroprusside** is the most effective drug and may reduce MR by up to 50% [152]. GTN is also strongly recommended [347, 352].
• Control of fast AF / cardioversion in case of new onset AF [347].

- Chronic MR: Diuretics and ACE-inhibitors [346]. Quinalapril improves the clinical situation and reduces the volume of regurgitation [353]. It has not been clarified whether this is a class effect (all available ACE-inhibitors) or not.

## b)    Mitral stenosis

MS does not develop acutely [347]. The main cause is rheumatic endocarditis. Vegetations are rare in cases of acute endocarditis. Myxoma of the atrium involving the valve (prolapsing into the valve area) or severe calcification of the annulus and the leaflets may provoke MS [347].

Main pathophysiology:
The pressure in the LA increases substantially [347]. There is left atrial hypertrophy and dilatation [346]. The filling of the LV depends increasingly on the active atrial contraction (active filling component of the LA). Each increase in heart rate with shortening of the diastole will lead to a further rise in left atrial pressure [346] and accompanying risk of pulmonary congestion or oedema [36, 347]. In the vast majority of cases a marked increase in heart rate (physical stress) and, in particular, new onset of AF will cause an acute decompensation [347].

Special therapeutic aspects:
- primary therapeutic aim is a reduction of the heart rate:
  Lengthening of diastole leads to:
  - Increase in LA filling volume with consecutive increase in LV-filling and thus SV,
  - a substantial decrease in pulmonary pressure [347].
Administer β-blockers or a Calcium-channel blocker such as Verapamil in order to slow down the heart rate, aim for a heart rate of 60–70 bpm [346, 347]. In certain conditions (duration of AF, size of LA, etc) cardioversion should be considered [354].
- Diuretics and/or nitrates will reduce left atrial pressure and will therefore relieve the symptoms of pulmonary congestion. However, caution should be used and low doses are preferred as diuretics or nitrates may reduce LV filling causing the CO/SV to drop [346].

## c)    Aortic regurgitation

The main causes of acute AR are acute bacterial endocarditis, chest trauma and aortic dissection [355, 356].

Main pathophysiology [347]:
In acute AR the LV is confronted by a rapid and substantial increase in filling volume causing a rapid rise in diastolic ventricular pressure. This pressure rise leads to an abnormally fast equalisation of the LV- and LA-pressure and premature closure of the mitral valve. Both effects may result in the development of pulmonary congestion/oedema [347] and the effective SV is reduced [347].
    The determinants of the regurgitation volume are the opening area (mostly fixed aortic valve), the duration of diastole (the longer the higher the regurgitation volume) and the diastolic transvalvular gradient [146]. Additionally, due to compensatory mechanisms the peripheral

vascular resistance will increase (afterload ↑), causing the regurgitant volume to increase further (ejection into the lower pressure compartment) [347]. Therefore, aim to avoid bradycardia and arterial hypertension [346, 347].

Special therapeutic aspects:
Vasodilators of the arterial vessels will reduce AR and enhance forward flow with redistribution of SV.

**Nitroprusside is the drug of choice in acute decompensated states** [357–359].

Good results can be achieved if using nifidepine [360] or ACE-inhibitors [361] in clinically stable situations. Vasodilators which affect mainly the venous system as well as diuretics will reduce preload, left-ventricular end-diastolic pressure and end-diastolic volume [357, 362]. Their effect is of symptom relief until valve replacement, which is needed in most cases, can be performed.

# d)     Aortic stenosis

Currently the main cause of AS is gradual valve calcification and degeneration, whereas previously a rheumatic background was common [363].

Main pathophysiology:
The **fixed** obstruction of the LVOT (due to AS) limits the output [38]. The pressure burden leads to LV hypertrophy and consecutively to an elevation of the LVEDP. Over time the contractility will be affected and LV dilatation will occur [347]. Psychological and physical stress may precipitate hypotension and syncope [346].
    Khot [364] recently suggested that, aside from the fixed valvular obstruction, the effective afterload affecting the LV exerts a systemic component as well: "Since the resistances in series are additive, the total resistance seen by the left ventricle is the sum of the resistance across the aortic valve plus the systemic vascular resistance. Therefore, increasing or decreasing systemic vascular resistance directly leads to proportional changes in the effective afterload of the left ventricle, even when there is severe aortic stenosis [365, 366]" – just as it is in conventional heart failure.

Special therapeutic aspects:
The conservative treatment options are very limited and all therapeutic measures run the risk of inducing haemodynamic deterioration [347]. Each therapeutic intervention should be initiated with caution.
• In case of acute decompensation **and** evidence of LV-dysfunction (as a component of ↑↑↑ afterload) vasodilators are indicated: **Nitroprusside** can be considered but **GTN** is probably preferable as it reduces afterload and blood pressure less aggressively than nitroprusside [364].
    Classically GTN and other vasodilators have been avoided in the treatment of acute heart failure due to decompensated severe aortic stenosis, but, as mentioned above, Khot [364] showed improved outcomes of the acute situation with faster resolution of pulmonary oedema and stabilisation of BP.

- GTN reduces the increased filling pressures and so will relieve dyspnoea in cases of pulmonary congestion or oedema [346, 347]. Diuretics (in low dosage) improve the symptoms of pulmonary congestion, but can induce hypovolaemia with a further drop in CO [368].
- Of special importance is the maintenance of sinus rhythm in order to retain the atrial component of LV filling, which now plays an important role in haemodynamic stability [348, 367]. Cardioversion should be considered in cases of new onset AF [347]. β-blockers or calcium-channel blockers should be titrated cautiously, aiming to lower the heart rate to at least 110 bpm or less [346, 347].

## 2.8    Summary

The most common underlying cause of heart failure is CAD, followed in Europe by hypertension and valvular disease [9–13]. Of patients with an AHFS, acute decompensation of chronic heart failure is the reason for hospital admission in the vast majority (60–75%) [6, 9].

The diagnosis is based on the patient's history and clinical examination [2, 81, 82] but echocardiography is a highly desirable additional diagnostic tool. It can decisively confirm the diagnosis and may be essential in identifying potentially reversible causes [2, 84].

Nevertheless, to diagnose acute heart failure may be difficult (non-specific symptoms, insensitive physical findings [76, 86]); thus an invasive haemodynamic assessment (as shown by Cotter [5]) of patients with signs of acute failure may be necessary in the diagnostic process [5].

AHFS are classified by the ESC in to six distinct clinical and haemodynamic entities [2] which govern the optimal therapeutic strategy.

The fundamental underlying pathophysiology is a progressive vasoconstriction. A vicious cycle of after-load mismatch ensues, with significantly reduced SV and markedly increased LVEDP, the latter potentially triggering development of pulmonary oedema [5, 7, 26–28, 30–32, 35–37].

The patient's clinical course and, at least, short term prognosis depends decisively upon the value of the sBP and the BUN concentration on admission [13, 70–72]. The vast majority of patients have a sBP of > 104 mm Hg on admission [6, 9, 23, 72], but a sBP < 120 mm Hg should give rise to concerns and consideration of critical care admission [6, 70, 72].

The principle therapeutic approach aims to reduce the LV-afterload along with the LVEDP [5, 28, 30, 58, 64, 72, 128–130, 136]. Early administration of intravenous vasodilators such as GTN/nesiritide or nitroprusside along with low doses of diuretics is essential [30, 134, 135, 135, 152].

Inotropic support should be avoided if possible, due to potentially harmful effects and a negative impact on outcome. This is particularly true where there is reasonably preserved systolic LV function (EF > 40%) and in clinically stable conditions [115, 120, 126, 136, 175–177, 193, 218, 248]. Inotropic agents are only indicated in patients with significantly impaired systolic function with impending cardiogenic shock refractory to vasodilators and diuretics and those in a life threatening situation [5, 70, 117, 120, 136, 152, 190, 250]. If catecholamine support is essential, dobutamine or levosimendan and noradrenaline should be preferred to dopamine and adrenaline, due to significantly lower mortality [289].

# Chapter 3

## Cardiogenic shock

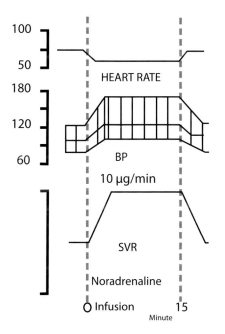

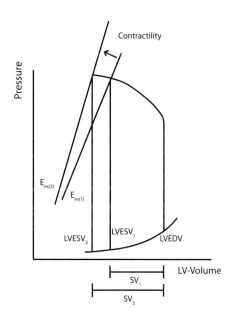

Left: Modified from Allwood, MJ *Br Med Bull* 19 (1963): 132;
Right: Modified from Opie, LH In: Braunwald, E *Heart Disease* 5th ed, WB Saunders Company, Philadelphia, 1997, p. 383.

## 3.1    Definition

**Shock** is defined as the maximal variant of dysregulation of the sophisticated regulatory systems of the organism due to a harmful event [1]. Central to this description we find a systemic derangement in perfusion (hypoperfusion) secondary to the critical decrease in cardiac output: There is an inadequate CO in respect to the patient's requirements, with disturbed microcirculation and insufficient supply of the tissues and organ systems causing widespread cellular hypoxia and vital organ dysfunction [1].

**Cardiogenic shock (CS)** [2] describes a **severe primarily myocardial dysfunction** with systemic hypocirculation / inadequate tissue perfusion (global tissue hypoxia) in the setting of adequate vascular volume [3] – and cellular as well as multi-organ dysfunction or failure [2, 4].

The US shock trial defines cardiogenic shock as [5]:

**Hypotension** with a systolic blood pressure < 90 mm Hg lasting ≥ 30 minutes

or

the necessity for catecholamines and/or rather IABP in order to maintain sufficient circulation with a sBP ≥ 90 mm Hg

and

**hypoperfusion** of the end organs due to the severely impaired cardiac performance, clinically characterised by cold peripheries (forearms and/or lower legs [6, 7]), disturbance of consciousness (altered mental status [8]) and oliguria (< 30 mls/h),

**hemodynamically**

described by CI ≤ 2.2 l/min/m² as well as PCWP ≥ 15 mm Hg (or pulmonary congestion on chest X-ray).

Menon [3] strongly recommends diagnosing CS in all patients exhibiting signs of inadequate tissue perfusion in the setting of severe cardiac dysfunction irrespective of the BP, **non-hypotensive** [9] or **pre-shock** [3, 10].

## 3.2    Epidemiology

Studies from unselected populations report an overall incidence of CS as 7.1% [11]. In the vast majority (> 75%) CS develops secondary to myocardial ischaemia [11–13], either due to chronic [1, 14, 15] or acute [16–20] coronary artery disease. The incidence of CS complicating acute myocardial infarction is reported as between 5% and 10% [11, 16–23]. LV-dysfunction is the main reason for the development of cardiogenic shock even in patients not suffering from CAD and thus not a result of ischaemia [24, 25].

The shock register and trial [26, 27] revealed that:

74.5%    CS was due to predominant LV-heart failure,
 8.3%    due to acute MR,

4.6%   due to ventricular septal rupture,
3.4%   were isolated right heart shock situations,
1.7%   were induced by tamponade or cardiac rupture,
3.0%   due to other reasons.

The overall in-hospital mortality is still high at approximately 60% [12].

CS is more likely to develop in the elderly [28–31], diabetic [28–31] patients suffering from acute anterior myocardial infarction [26–31], patients with a history of previous infarction(s) [30, 31], patients with peripheral vascular disease [30, 31] and patients with cerebrovascular disease [30, 31].

CS often develops over hours, the shock trial [26] as well as other publications [19, 32, 33] found that 75% of all shock states developed within 24 hours of presentation, and in the GUSTO-study [16, 23] it was even higher at 89%.

## 3.3   Aetiology

The most common causes of cardiogenic shock are [12, 34–36]:
- acute impairment of **myocardial** pump function from:
  - acute myocardial infarction and associated complications, including rupture of a papillary muscle or septum, severe MR and pericardial tamponade,
  - acute myocarditis,
  - intoxication with negatively inotropic drugs,
  - myocardial contusion,
  - sepsis and septic shock.
- acute valvular disease (AR or MR due to endocarditis, aortic dissection or chordae rupture) / acute exacerbation of a chronic valvular disease,
- acute decompensated chronic heart failure, particularly end-stage cardiomyopathy,
- acute right heart failure (right ventricular myocardial infarction; acute, severe broncho-pulmonary diseases),
- persistent severe rhythm disturbances,
- acute decompensation of hypertrophic cardiomyopathy (i.e. due to acute atrial fibrillation),
- left atrial myxoma.

## 3.4   Pathophysiological aspects and special features

### a)   Classical pathophysiology and new CS paradigm

In cardiogenic shock the overwhelming majority of cases are caused by an **abrupt depression** and/or **loss of contractility** (intrinsic performance) of the heart irrespective of loading conditions with a **subsequent significant fall in SV/CO** [1, 2, 5, 36].

This occurs most often due to a critical loss of contractile tissue/mass [36] secondary to acute myocardial infarction [16–18, 21, 22] with **acute loss of total pump force** [37] and an additional reduction of the ventricular compliance [38]. Hence, **in CS both systolic and diasto-**

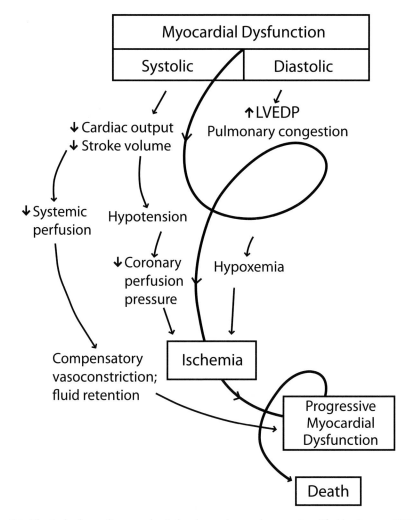

**Figure 3.1** Classic shock paradigm, mechanical and neurohumoral aspects (modified by Antman [41]).

**lic function are failing** [39, 40]. Traditionally, CS is seen as a mechanical problem [36] with corresponding humoral activation and response [39, 41]; this paradigm is summarised in the diagram (see Figure 3.1) by Antman [41] who confirmed work by Califf [39].

As stated, severe myocardial dysfunction, as in the case of CS, leads directly to both decreased SV and an increase in LVEDP [36, 39, 40]. Subsequently, the **marked reduction in SV causes hypotension** [36] and **systemic hypoperfusion** [36], compromising the coronary perfusion, causing myocardial ischaemia or aggravating existing myocardial ischaemia [5, 39, 41, 42] with progressive impairment of myocardial function as the result [5, 39, 41, 42]. Furthermore, as depicted by the diagram above, in response to the considerable impairment of the cardiac contractility [15, 36, 42, 43] a **compensatory systemic vasoconstriction** [36, 39, 41–43] secondary to neuro-endocrine [36, 42–44], in particular sympathetic activation [36, 39, 41–43], **and**

**fluid retention** [42, 44] occur. The systemic vasoconstriction and the fluid load exert additional adverse loading conditions [41–43, 45] (particularly increasing afterload [42, 43, 45, 46]) onto the already compromised myocardial function.

However, surprisingly, several studies in **cardiogenic shock** [5, 47–51] have revealed **a fundamentally different haemodynamic profile** than expected and previously established:

Although the contractility is severely impaired with a marked fall in SV and a compromised diastolic function **the peripheral systemic resistance** is only **marginally to moderately elevated.** This **inappropriate vasoconstriction** (inappropriate low systemic vascular resistance) in relation to the severity of the myocardial depression found in the majority of patients [50–53] reflects a **systemic inflammatory reaction (SIRS) to be present in CS** [5, 12, 47–49, 54–59].

Reperfusion induces the release of vasodilatatory acting mediators [56, 60] and Kohsaka [53] detected high levels of inducible NO-synthetase subsequent to the release of inflammatory mediators in patients with acute myocardial infarction. Concomitant, high concentrations of NO and peroxy-nitrates (mediators with vasodilative effects) counterbalance the initially induced compensatory vasoconstriction and, in fact, lead to an inappropriate circulatory response with vasodilation [5, 9, 50–52, 56, 58, 59]. Furthermore, low peripheral resistance predisposes patients with CS to endothelial damage [53]. So, the systemic inflammatory reaction contributes substantially to the pathogenesis and the course of CS with **further reduction of myocardial**

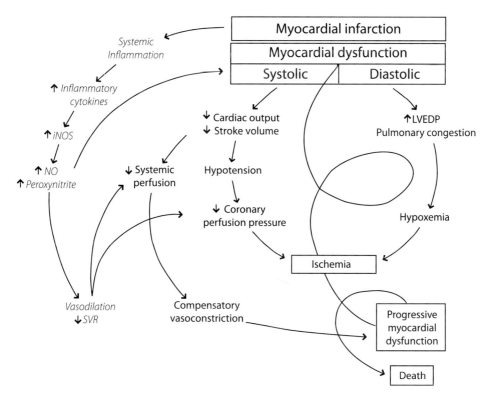

**Figure 3.2** Right side: classic shock paradigm, mechanical and neurohumoral aspects; left side and in italics: influence of the inflammatory response syndrome: New cardiogenic shock paradigm by Hochman [48].

**contractility** secondary to the release of vasodilative (may cause further ischaemia) and **myocardial depressive mediators** [40, 61–65]. This may lead to profound, persistent and refractory vasodilatation and hypotension [1, 48, 56, 59] and to the development of MODS/MOF [5, 48, 49] with its deleterious outcome, if not treated adequately and in time [1, 48, 66].

This 'only' **marginal to moderate increase in afterload in the initial phase** has proved to be **pathognomonic of CS** [47–49, 51].

A small group of patients in the SHOCK registry and trial [5, 26, 27] were clinically normotensive or only mildly hypotensive but still diagnosed as cardiogenic shock: They were systemically hypoperfused with low CO and elevated left ventricular filling pressures but with an elevated SVR and therefore able to maintain a reasonable blood pressure [9]. These patients should perhaps have been classified as being in a pre-shock state [3], where the systemic inflammatory response is not yet significantly activated.

Hochman [48] suggested a new cardiogenic shock paradigm, having integrating the newer pathophysiological aspects [49, 57] within the older existing concepts [41] as depicted in Figure 3.2.

## b)    The role and impact of hypotension in CS

Myocardial perfusion is compromised by hypotension [5, 42] and may induce ischaemia or exacerbate existing ischaemia [36]. The decreased coronary perfusion pressure (especially in multivessel coronary disease [39]) secondary to the decrease in MAP, caused by the poor cardiac performance/contractility and vasodilatation, may lead to a critically low BP [5, 39, 41, 49]. Critical hypoperfusion itself aggravates the myocardial perfusion deficit [63], exacerbating the myocardial ischaemia and implementing a vicious cycle leading to a more and more severely ischaemic myocardium [39, 41]. This is seen even in shock states not initially caused by impaired **myo**cardial contractility [1, 2] when the blood pressure is so low that the perfusion of the end-organs [1, 13] (especially the heart [13, 57, 67–69]) becomes critically dependent on the haemodynamics [5, 39, 69, 70].

## c)    Myocardial ischaemia and LV-compliance

The compliance of the left ventricle will be reduced by myocardial ischaemia, and subsequently the LVEDP will rise [71–75] as will the pulmonary capillary pressure, putting the patient at risk of developing pulmonary oedema [73–75]. Additionally, LV end-diastolic filling increases in the situation of severely impaired systolic LV-function in order to maintain SV [36, 39, 76]; this will augment the LVEDP further, putting the patients at even higher risk of pulmonary congestion/oedema [39, 77] and further ischaemia [36, 39].

## d)     Other acute causes of a substantial impairment in contractility:

- Transient acute myocardial ischaemia [1, 15, 78] on a background of **chronic CAD** and the accompanying diastolic dysfunction [79–81] is able to induce an abrupt impairment of the contractility of viable myocardial tissue;
- Considerable **regurgitant flow** [1] from acute mitral insufficiency (**acute MR**) as a mechanical complication of acute myocardial infarction [12, 36], ischaemic MR [82–86], and mitral valve insufficiency subsequent to transient hypo-perfusion (ischaemia) in case of chronic CAD [87] can be responsible for a sudden decrease in SV/CO;
- **Acute AR** is most commonly caused by infective endocarditis [88]. The rapidity of occurrence of the regurgitant flow does not allow the establishment of any specific compensatory mechanisms (i.e. LV-dilatation) [89, 90]. Consequently the SV/CO (forward stroke volume) will significantly diminish as well as the LVEDP increasing [1];
- **Myocarditis** sometimes causes markedly impaired contractility and hence reduced forward flow [91, 92];
- **Drugs** may have negative inotropic potential and the ability to initiate the production and release of pro-inflammatory mediators from cardiomyocytes and other (haematological) cells which can promote the inflammatory process and be directly cardio-depressive [62, 80]. Even catecholamines (released as part of the compensatory mechanisms or administered as therapeutic agents) may induce the production of pro-inflammatory cytokines (i.e. Interleukin IL-6) and thus provide a further direct depression of contractility [80, 93, 94].

## 3.5     Clinical features and diagnostic remarks

## a)     Hypoperfusion

In the vast majority the **diagnosis of CS** is established by **clinical signs of hypoperfusion, ischaemic chest pain, enzymatic analysis and ECG** [95]. A normal ECG virtually excludes the possibility of CS caused by myocardial infarction [39]. In addition, an echocardiogram is absolutely essential in the initial assessment of all patients suffering from (cardiogenic) shock [3, 36, 96–98] and should be performed as early as possible.

The **crucial aspect** in the **diagnosis of CS** is the identification of **hypoperfusion** in the **setting of considerable cardiac dysfunction** [1, 3, 5, 36, 39]. The following signs and features are suggestive of organ / tissue hypoperfusion [3, 5, 36, 95, 99, 100]:

- pallor, ashen grey or cyanotic skin,
- cold peripheries (forearms and/or lower legs [6]), cold skin, moist and clammy, mottled extremities,
- altered mental status [8]: quiet, apathetic patient, sometimes restless, apprehensive or confused,
- reduced urine production/oliguria, < 30 ml/h or < 0.5 ml/kg/h for ≥ 2 h [100],
- thready pulse of poor quality,
- arterial hypotension.

CS should be considered in all patients presenting with unexplained hypotension and/or low cardiac output, unexplained impairment of mental function and unexplained pulmonary congestion [5, 13, 36]. In fact Menon [3, 9, 10] strongly recommends **diagnosing CS** in all patients exhibiting **signs of inadequate tissue perfusion** in the setting of **severe cardiac dysfunction irrespective of the BP.**

"CS is diagnosed after documentation of myocardial dysfunction and exclusion of alternative causes of hypotension like hypovolaemia, haemorrhage, sepsis, pulmonary embolism, tamponade, aortic dissection and pre-existing valvular disease" [36].

Ander [101] expresses doubts that clinical signs are sensitive enough to detect occult cardiogenic shock, particularly in patients with congestive heart failure because clinical signs may fail to diagnose inadequate oxygen delivery [102–105]; thus, the measurement of $ScvO_2$ and serum lactate are recommended [101, 106]:

A lactate > 2 mmol/l together with a $ScvO_2$ < 60% ($SvO_2$ < 65%) suggests occult shock [101].

Sixty-four percent of all patients included in the US shock register presented with hypotension, evidence of ineffective CO/hypoperfusion and pulmonary congestion [8], but 28% had evidence of peripheral hypoperfusion and hypotension and **did not** suffer from pulmonary congestion [8]. Thus, clear lungs may still be present even with elevated PCWP and CS [8]. This phenomenon (elevated PCWP but no clinical or radiological signs of pulmonary congestion) has been described previously [107]; it deserves emphasis because administration of large amounts of fluid will be deleterious [8, 108]. Do not treat these patients with large boluses of fluid [3, 108].

The timely identification of patients in a pre-shock [3, 10] or non-hypotensive shock [9] state is of special value to allow therapeutic intervention and prevent decline. Clinical signs of hypoperfusion (in particular cold, clammy skin and oliguria) are strongly associated with increased mortality, independent of blood pressure and other haemodynamic parameters [109]. Hypoperfusion may be a marker of impending haemodynamic collapse [9] and **tachycardia** in this setting (HR > 90/min) should be interpreted as a pre-shock symptom and not as a response to low cardiac output and subsequent increased sympathetic tone [3]. Take care particularly in patients with anterior AMI and keep in mind that up to 30% of patients with AMI develop cardiogenic shock late (day 5) in their disease course – and with a very poor prognosis [110].

In this situation the choice of medication should be made carefully. The use of β-blockers, in general indicated and life-saving in AMI [111, 112], may precipitate shock development in these patients [3, 12, 67, 113]. Additionally, the possible life saving compensatory activation of the renin-angiotensin system should not be counteracted by administration of ACE-inhibitors [114, 115].

## b)     Right ventricular infarction

A significant **infarction of the right ventricle** (RV-AMI) complicates 50% of all inferior myocardial infarctions [116]. On an ECG, ST-elevation in $V_{R3}$ and/or $V_{R4}$ (right praecordial leads) in patients with inferior ST-elevation acute myocardial infarction is specific for RV-ischaemia due to a proximal RCA-lesion [117]. Predominantly the inferior and posterior parts of the RV are involved [118].

The haemodynamic alterations and the severity of circulatory compromise are determined by the damage of the RV itself (extent of RV ischaemia and the subsequent RV-dysfunction), the ventricular interaction (mediated by the septum and by the restraining pericardium [117] affecting the LV-function) and the involvement of the LV in the ischaemic injury [118]. Furthermore, the RV is only able to compensate in a very limited manner for acute increases in afterload or volume [119–122]. Hence, rapid haemodynamic compromise and early onset of hypotension and shock occur [119]. On the other hand, a sufficient RV pump function is necessary to prevent LV pump failure – series effect [123, 124] – ensuring the delivery of an appropriate preload required to guarantee LV output [123–125].

The LV may assist the RV to generate the force needed by contributing to the septal contraction [126–128]. A loss of this support due to LV infarction, in particular if the septum is involved, could induce further circulatory deterioration [126–130]. Hence, the critical interaction between both ventricles may considerably affect the haemodynamics recognised in RV-AMI with the RV as a crucial component responsible for the development for CS [131].

The recognition of this special issue is important due to the special treatment needs: well balanced and monitored fluid administration, fluid restriction in case of manifest RV-failure, and CS [131–134], preservation of AV-synchrony and reduction of increased RV-afterload [135–137].

## c) The LVEDP in cardiogenic shock

The LVEDP and its measurement in the definition and diagnosis of cardiogenic shock should be assessed critically; an elevated LVEDP may not be a sensitive or specific parameter with which to diagnose CS:

- Acute severe heart failure is not necessarily accompanied by high LV-filling pressures. Some patients will definitely have normal or even low LVEDP's [8, 138–140];
- The LVEDP (PCWP) does not reflect the amount of extravascular lung water [141–143] due to cardiac dysfunction in a uniform way [139, 141–143];
- An abnormally high LVEDP ($\geq 15$ mm Hg as described in the definition) may only reflect an abnormal stiffness of the LV [144] (impaired LV-compliance, i.e. due to ischaemia [71, 72]). It is well known that, particularly in critically ill patients, the compliance of the ventricles continuously varies, contributing to the heterogeneous response and changes of the LVEDP value [145–148]. Even in healthy persons absolutely no correlation was found between changes in ventricular filling and the change in value of LVEDP [149];
- The PCWP (as well as the CVP) does not adequately represent the pre-load or intravascular volume status and its changes in volume loading or unloading, either in healthy subjects [149] or in the critically ill [146, 150].

Thus, no reasonable correlation between LVEDV and LVEDP could ever be established [146, 149, 150] and in preference, the transmural LVEDP may be helpful to guide and monitor disease and therapeutic measures [151]. For further details see Chapter 1, paragraph 3b.

Table 3.1 Clinical Presentation and Haemodynamic Characteristics of Cardiogenic Pre-shock and Manifest Shock

| WARM and DRY | COLD and DRY | WARM and WET | COLD and WET |
|---|---|---|---|
| | **28% of all CS patients**<br><br>Clinically often surprisingly stable or otherwise dominated by symptoms of hypoperfusion (see right panel).<br><br>**Haemodynamics:** sBP ↓/↓↓↓ (<90 mmHg for ≥30 min or catecholamines required);<br><br>CI ↓/↓↓↓ (CI ≤ 2.2 l/min/m²); no pulmonary congestion and often with a normal PCWP, **hypoperfusion:** mild to severe.<br><br>**Performance of an echocardiogram is vital.**<br><br>CS should be considered in all patients presenting with unexplained hypotension or low cardiac output and unexplained altered consciousness, irrespective of BP.<br><br>**Pre-shock criteria,** see right panel<br><br>**Clinical scenarios most likely in this group:** ESC 4a, 4b and ESC- 6 | | **64% of CS patients**<br><br>Clinically dominated by symptoms of hypoperfusion: pallor, ashen grey or cyanotic skin, cold peripheries, thready pulse, altered mental status, oliguria (<30 ml/h), arterial hypotension and pulmonary congestion; auscultated $S_3$.<br><br>**Haemodynamics:** sBP ↓/↓↓↓ (<90 mmHg for ≥30 min or catecholamines required);<br><br>CI ↓/↓↓↓ (CI ≤ 2.2 l/min/m²): PCWP ↑/↑↑↑ (≥15 mmHg or pulmonary congestion on chest x-ray); **hypoperfusion:** mild to severe<br><br>**Performance of an echocardiogram is vital.**<br><br>CS should be considered in all patients presenting with unexplained hypotension or low cardiac output, pulmonary congestion and unexplained altered consciousness, irrespective of BP.<br><br>**Pre-shock criteria:** signs of inadequate tissue perfusion in the setting of severe cardiac dysfunction irrespective of the BP. Often a history of AMI, a cold and clammy patient with tachycardia and crackles ≥ 50% of total lung area suggesting pulmonary oedema.<br><br>**Clinical scenarios most likely in this group:** ESC 4a, 4b and pre-shock.. |

## d)     Differential diagnosis of cardiogenic shock [3, 39, 95]

- hypovolaemic shock,
- dissection of the aorta,
- pulmonary embolism,
- bacteraemia,
- neurogenic shock,
- anaphylactic shock,
- Takotsubo syndrome [152, 153].

## 3.6    Therapy

A substantial number of publications have addressed the best therapeutic approach to CS complicating AMI – the most likely scenario in the vast majority of patients with CS [5, 67, 154–161].

Both retrospective [67, 154–158] and prospective randomised controlled trials [5, 159, 160] have produced considerable evidence that an invasive approach (emergency revascularisation by PCI/operation with and without prior thrombolytic therapy) is beneficial. The effect was similar for both manifest CS at admission and in the event of delayed onset [162]. The hospital mortality could be reduced from 75% (occluded vessel) to 33% (re-opened vessel by PCI) [161, 163, 164,]. When emergency revascularisation was combined with and supported by IABP, the benefit was even more profound with an absolute mortality reduction of 13% after one year follow-up as compared to medical treatment alone [159]. The use of IABP with thrombolytic treatment has also shown substantial benefit [32].

## a)     Main therapeutic strategies:

- Coronary intervention in acute coronary syndromes [5, 26, 39, 48, 70, 154–161, 165]. This comprises thrombolytic therapy, PCI, rescue – PCI, or emergency CABG,
- Emergency operation for mechanical complications following acute myocardial infarction (rupture of the septum, acute MR, etc) [166, 167],
- Emergency valve replacement/repair in case of acute/acutely decompensated AR or MR [168, 169],
- Emergency operation for acute ascending aortic dissection [168, 169],
- Pericardial puncture/drainage if pericardial tamponade (traumatic or inflammatory) is the reason for shock [168, 169],
- Thrombolysis/thrombus fragmentation/operation in case of acute fulminant pulmonary embolism [168, 169],
- Adequate treatment of rhythm disturbances if they are the main reason for shock: Temporary pacemaker in bradycardia [170], DC cardioversion, emergency ablation or anti-arrhythmic medication (Amiodarone) in case of sustained VT [168, 169], magnesium in case of torsade de pointe tachycardia [171–173].
- Immediate pleural drainage in tension pneumothorax [174].

## b)        Adjunctive treatment

### i)        Re-establishing and maintaining appropriate coronary and systemic perfusion

Critical hypoperfusion reduces the myocardial perfusion or aggravates an already present myo-cardial perfusion deficit [63]. Persistent myocardial ischaemia and hypoperfusion will cause a vicious cycle leading to an increasingly ischaemic myocardium [39, 41]. The perfusion of the end-organs [1, 13] (especially the heart [13, 57, 67–69]) becomes critically dependent on the haemodynamics [5, 69, 70].

In order to provide an appropriate coronary perfusion pressure in patients with IHD, avoid-ing (further) ischaemia, and preventing the intact myocardium from hypoperfusion, a MAP ≥ 70(75) – 80 mm Hg [175–178] should be sufficient. In patients with other reasons for CS, such as acute myocarditis, a MAP ≥ 65 mm Hg may suffice [178, 179]. Guidelines recommend keeping the sBP ≥ 100 mm Hg in case of CS, but no studies are available to substantially sup-port this value [180].

Furthermore, although a higher perfusion pressure does not automatically improve tissue perfusion, in the case of the heart there is evidence that an increase in systemic and hence coro-nary perfusion pressure indeed means an improvement in the tissue perfusion. Both, Vlahakes [181] and Di Giantomasso [182] found a significant increase in myocardial tissue perfusion while administering noradrenaline to treat hypotension, increasing the systemic as well as the coronary perfusion pressure.

### ii)        Fluid administration

In life-threatening situations with severe hypotension and tissue hypoperfusion, a fluid chal-lenge as described by Vincent and Weil [183] is justifiable, even in cases of cardiogenic shock [8, 184]. But remember that only 10–15% of all patients with CS suffer from a relative or absolute volume deficit needed in order to benefit from fluid loading [185], although, understandably, Hunt [184] demands that a **confirmed volume deficit** be treated before commencing any other measures. However, as Michard has shown, in the case of severely impaired contractility no significant increase in SV and blood pressure can be expected by volume loading [150]. Thus, close monitoring and a careful assessment are essential in order to avoid volume overloading with its harmful consequences [186].

### iii)       Vasopressor administration

In critical hypoperfusion, meanwhile, noradrenaline (NA) is the preferred drug: When com-pared to dopamine, it shows an improvement of renal and myocardial tissue perfusion [181, 182, 187–189], and within reasonable dose ranges no unfavourable effects on mucosa/gut or thyroid perfusion [190–194] are expected. Sakr found that administration of dopamine or adrenaline was associated with a significantly higher mortality when compared to dobutamine and noradrenaline [195].

However, dopamine is still recommended in guidelines as the first-choice drug in cardio-genic shock situations when systolic pressure ranges between 70 and 90 mm Hg [70, 196, 197]. Further NA should be administered or added in the event of systolic pressures < 70 mm Hg or if dopamine dosages > 20 µg/kg/min are required [57, 70, 196, 198].

**iv)**     **Intra-aortic balloon counter pulsation**

Califf [39] sees IABP as a standard component in the therapy of CS. **IABP** provides effective haemodynamic support and, of extreme importance, **increases the coronary blood flow**. In particular, **IABP is efficacious in the initial stabilisation** of patients suffering from CS [199–203]. IABP improves outcome [200–202] and shows at least a trend towards lower mortality even when used alone [16, 26, 203]. Unfortunately, IABP is still underused [3].

Main IABP effects include [32, 42, 203–205]:
- afterload ↓,
- ↑ diastolic coronary perfusion pressure,
- ↑ CO,
- ↑ coronary blood flow.

The recommended indications (evidence class I, level B) for IABP [70, 206–209] are:
- medically refractory CS complicating AMI [206, 209], particularly prior to any required transfer [3],
- post cardiac surgery,
- refractory angina,
- other reasons for CS including refractory malignant ventricular arrhythmias [210],
- severe MR [209] or ventricular septal rupture [209].

**v)**     **Inotropic medication**

As mentioned in Chapter 2, inotropic drugs are traditionally used to increase CO (SV) and improve peripheral and vital organ perfusion [211, 212] in low output situations which may be life threatening [51, 68, 70, 197].

A combination of **Dopamine** and **Dobutamine** is still recommended as being the gold standard in the treatment of cardiogenic shock [37, 57, 70, 197, 213, 214]. As long as the systolic blood pressure is not less than 80–85 mm Hg or stabilised on that level by administrating a reasonable dose of dopamine (< 15–20 µg/kg/min), dobutamine can and should be added [70, 214]. Due to the favourable effects of noradrenaline discussed above more recent publications prefer the combination of dobutamine and noradrenaline, once a systolic blood pressure > 85(90) mm Hg is achieved and maintained [69, 215]. NA is indicated as well (instead of dopamine or additional to dopamine) if the initial sBP is < 70 mm Hg, or if a sBP of 85–90 mm Hg, despite dopamine infusion (dosage not > 20 µg/kg/min), cannot be achieved [70, 191, 197, 216].

In the event of a reasonable BP (Ryan [191] suggests sBP ≥ 90 mm Hg) or in pre-shock situations with a sBP ≥ 90 mm Hg, dobutamine is still validated as the first choice drug when aiming to support and improve the contractility and thus tissue perfusion [1, 39, 57, 70, 197, 214]. However, as mentioned, there is growing and clear evidence of adverse events and increased mortality when using inotropic agents [198, 213, 217–219].

Phosphodiesterase-inhibitors do not have any benefits when compared to dobutamine, with the exception that they are effective in patients who are on regular β-blocker medication, and patients do not develop tolerance as with dobutamine [215, 220].

The relatively new **Levosimendan**, a calcium sensitising agent, has shown very encouraging results in the treatment of severe heart failure [221–225]. Some studies found a significantly lower mortality when compared to dobutamine in patients treated for AHFS [222–226]. Levosimendan not only has favourable effects on systolic function but, in contrast to dobutamine, the diastolic function substantially improves as well (no adverse influence on relaxation) [227–230]. Furthermore, there is a considerable beneficial impact on the failing right ventricle [231–234]. Unfortunately, the recently published SURVIVE-study [235] could only demonstrate favourable effects of levosimendan compared to dobutamine in subgroups (acute exacerbated chronic heart failure) [236]. The RUSSLAN-study did find a substantial benefit for patients suffering from heart failure as a complication of AMI when treated with levosimendan rather than dobutamine [223].

Levosimendan can be used instead of dobutamine as a positively inotropic drug in CS unless the systolic blood pressure is less than 85 mm Hg [231, 237, 238], in which case a combination with noradrenaline may be used as some authors recommend [231, 239–241].

As mentioned previously, an aggravation of hypotension and hypoperfusion may be fatal and should be avoided [36, 39, 41, 63, 67–70]. Restoration of normovolaemia and omitting the loading dose are measures which will avoid hypoperfusion secondary to levosimendan administration [69, 237, 238].

## c)     The systemic inflammatory reaction

As detailed above, a systemic inflammatory reaction occurs not only in septic shock but also in cardiogenic shock [48, 49, 54–59]. Keh [242] showed that hydrocortisone produced a beneficial effect on the inflammatory response in patients with septic shock whilst, Annane [243] administered hydrocortisone and fludrocortisone, producing a lower mortality, probably due to treating the relative adrenal insufficiency. Steroid use is now recommended in critically ill patients with septic shock [244]. On this background Confalonieri [245] showed that patients suffering from community-acquired pneumonia with severe systemic inflammatory reaction benefited considerably when treated with low dose hydrocortisone, with a reduction in hospital stay and mortality. This has also been found to be valid for patients with systemic inflammatory response following cardiothoracic operations [246]. Hence, there may be a role for low dose hydrocortisone (200–300 mg/day) in case of therapy-resistant [247, 248] cardiogenic shock, although this has yet to be validated in large studies.

## d)     Renal function

Renal dysfunction is known to accompany acute heart failure syndromes in a substantial number of cases [249–251]; if present, patient prognosis is poor [251, 252]. It is not only the direct influence of the impaired cardiac function affecting the kidneys but neurohumoral activation may also indirectly compromise the renal function [253, 254]. The so-called 'vasomotor nephropathy' is a transient, partly or completely reversible renal dysfunction resulting from vasoconstriction of the afferent arteriole caused by the abnormal haemodynamics and/or neurohumoral activation [253, 254].

Therefore, shortly following restoration of an appropriate circulation attention should be directed to the renal function [255, 256]. The main prerequisites are eu/normovolaemia and an adequate perfusion pressure (MAP ≥ 70–80 mm Hg) [189, 255, 257].

If an adequate diuresis does not commence spontaneously after volume status and blood pressure are optimised, **one** attempt to induce diuresis by administration of diuretics (bolus application) appears to be reasonable [255, 258]. If this is ineffective and there is persistent oligo/anuria or increasing (> 1.5–2.0 of baseline level) serum creatinine levels signalling acute kidney injury [259] and a poor prognosis [260], then options include a furosemide infusion [261], bumetanide [262] or a combination of furosemide and metolazone [263]. However, recurrent unsuccessful attempts with diuretics are likely to be harmful [264–266].

So, in the face of ongoing oligo/anuria early consideration should be made of **CRRT**, continuous renal replacement therapy. CRRT has a 'neutral haemodynamic behaviour' with only a **minimal effect on MAP** [256, 257], which is essential, especially in the case of fluid overload [256]. Continuous renal replacement therapy also eliminates cardiopulmonary toxic substances and, most relevantly, myocardial depressant factors [267].

## e)     Compensation of acidosis

In shock states metabolic acidosis occurs due to elevated serum lactate in response to peripheral hypoperfusion [268]. Buffering should only be considered if the pH < 7.1 or it is evident that the vasopressor or inotropic medications are not effective due to the low pH, and one should aim to raise the pH only moderately, not exceeding a target pH of 7.2–7.25. The decision to use buffer agents is controversial [269–272] and some authors refuse to do so [273]. There exists very little evidence as to beneficial effects of buffer agents [274]; however if buffering is necessary, on current evidence tromethamine should be the preferred drug [275–277], as it has less side effects than bicarbonate solutions.

In mechanically ventilated patients mild hyperventilation is a nimble tool to remove excess acid in the form of carbon dioxide [278, 279].

## f)     Anticoagulation therapy

Patients with cardiogenic shock should be anticoagulated in order to avoid disseminated intravascular coagulation (DIC) or thrombo-embolic events [280–283]. Although lacking definitive studies, intravenous (to avoid inadequate absorption in peripheral hypoperfusion) administration of 500–800 IU/h unfractionated heparin is generally recommended [280]. Prophylaxis of thromboembolism may be achieved either by 5000 IU of unfractionated heparin three times a day, or an adequate dose of low molecular weight heparin [283, 284].

## 3.7     Summary

Cardiogenic shock is characterised by global tissue hypoxia and vital organ dysfunction secondary to **severe, myocardial dysfunction** with systemic hypocirculation [1, 2].

Characteristic clinical signs of hypoperfusion are cold, mottled, and clammy peripheries [6, 7], altered mental status [8], oliguria (< 30 ml/h) and pulmonary congestion. Arterial hypoten-

**Table 3.2** Cardiogenic Shock, Treatment Regimes

## WARM and DRY / COLD and DRY

**Haemodynamic monitoring essential**

**Treat underlying disease**

**Intravenous fluids:** strictly monitored, dynamic tests of fluid responsiveness [289–293]; fluid challenge in life threatening situations only.

| sBP < 70 mm Hg | sBP ≥ 70–(90)100 mm Hg | | | sBP ≥ (90)100 mm Hg | | | |
|---|---|---|---|---|---|---|---|
| SVR ↓/n | SVR ↑-↑↑ | EF ≤ 0.4 CPI ≤ 0.3 | EF > 0.4 CPI > 0.3 | SVR n/↑ | SVR ↑-↑↑ | EF ≤ 0.4 CPI ≤ 0.3 | EF > 0.4 CPI > 0.3 |
| NA plus IABP add LEV/DOB if stabilised (BP N + SVR ↑-↑↑) | NA ± IABP | NA ± IABP add DOB/LEV if stabilised (BP N + SVR ↑-↑↑) | LEV/DOB – if BP↓ stop DOB/LEV ± add/ start NA | | | | Very low dose gtn – if BP ↓ stop gtn and start LEV/ DOB ± NA as appropriate |

**Loop diuretics** after haemodynamic stabilisation (MAP ≥ 70(75), sBP 100) **when clear evidence** of DVI.

**CRRT** if refractory to a reasonable attempt with drugs or in haemodynamically unstable patients[256, 257, 294].

In case of isolated or dominant right heart failure, see Chapter 4

## WARM and WET / COLD and WET

**Haemodynamic monitoring essential**

**Treat underlying disease**

In principle no IV fluids. Fluid challenge only in life threatening situations, otherwise fluid administration only if clear evidence of hypovolaemia with fluid responsiveness confirmed.

| sBP < 70 mm Hg | sBP ≥ 70–90(100) mm Hg | | | sBP ≥ 90(100) mm Hg | | | |
|---|---|---|---|---|---|---|---|
| SVR ↓/n | SVR ↑-↑↑ | EF ≤ 0.4 CPI ≤ 0.3 | EF > 0.4 CPI > 0.3 | SVR n/↑ | SVR ↑-↑↑ | EF ≤ 0.4 CPI ≤ 0.3 | EF > 0.4 CPI > 0.3 |
| NA plus IABP add LEV/DOB if stabilised (BP N + SVR ↑-↑↑) | NA ± IABP | NA ± IABP add DOB/ LEV if stabilised (BP N + SVR ↑-↑↑) | LEV/DOB – if BP↓ stop DOB/LEV ± add/ start NA as appropriate | | | | Very low dose gtn – if BP↓ stop gtn and start LEV/ DOB ± NA as appropriate |

**Loop diuretics** after haemodynamic stabilisation (and MAP ≥ 70(75), sBP ≥ 100) **when evidence** of fluid overload.

**CRRT early** if refractory to a reasonable attempt with drugs or in haemodynamically unstable patients[256, 257, 294].

sion (sBP < 90 mm Hg) although a criteria of CS [5], is not a decisive parameter and a sBP ≥ 90 mm Hg will not exclude the presence of non hypotensive or pre-shock [3, 9, 10]. CS should be considered in all patients exhibiting signs of inadequate tissue perfusion in the setting of severe cardiac dysfunction irrespective of the BP [3, 9, 10].

Acute or chronic myocardial ischaemia are the underlying aetiology [11, 12, 13, 36] in the vast majority (> 75%) of cases. CS complicates AMI in 5 and 10% of cases [11, 16–19, 21–23]. Other underlying aetiologies are valvular heart diseases, drugs with negative inotropic effects, and infections like acute myocarditis and sepsis [12, 34–36].

Pathophysiologically, the acute loss in pump force [37, 39] and the additional reduction in compliance (altered diastolic properties) [5, 38, 72] are traditionally expected to be compensated by marked neuro-endocrine [36, 42–44] and sympathetic activation [36, 39, 41, 42, 61] inducing compensatory fluid retention [42, 44] and **systemic vasoconstriction** [36, 39, 41–43]. However, in the majority of patients an inappropriate vasoconstriction (inappropriate low systemic vascular resistance/inappropriate compensation) in relation to the severity of the myocardial depression is found [50–53]. This reflects a **systemic inflammatory reaction (SIRS) present in CS** [5, 9, 12, 47–49, 54–59] which interferes with the usual compensatory mechanisms. An 'only' **marginal to moderate compensatory increase in systemic vascular resistance is therefore pathognomonic for CS** [5, 47–49, 51]. The new pathophysiological concept is described by Hochman [48].

In spite of all therapeutic improvements, the overall in-hospital mortality remains high at 60%.

Fundamental to therapeutic efforts stands reperfusion procedures in case of AMI [5, 67, 161]. The hospital mortality can be reduced from 75% to 33% by reopening an occluded vessel by PCI [161, 163, 164]. By combining emergency revascularisation with circulatory support from IABP, the benefit is even more profound with an absolute mortality reduction of 13% after one year of follow-up compared to medical treatment alone [159].

Critical hypoperfusion must be avoided and restoration of sufficient coronary perfusion is of vital importance [5, 39, 41, 63]. The use of vasopressor medication, preferably NA [187, 188, 285–287], aiming for a MAP between 70(75) and 80 mm Hg [175–178] and IABP [206–209, 200–202] will be essential, life saving measures [68, 70, 195, 288]. Inotropic drugs may be required and levosimendan is probably the preferred agent [68, 70, 213, 226, 235, 236, 239].

# Chapter 4

## Acute right heart failure

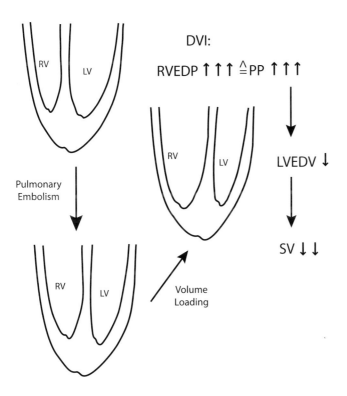

## 4.1    Definition

Acute **right heart failure** (RV-F) [overview by 1, 2] is defined by haemodynamic parameters and the haemodynamic behaviour of the right ventricle, but results in a reduced right ventricular stroke volume [3]:

$$\text{RVEDV} \uparrow - \uparrow\uparrow\uparrow \text{ and at the same time } \downarrow - \downarrow\downarrow\downarrow \text{ RV- EF, and RV-SV } \downarrow - \downarrow\downarrow\downarrow$$

**Right heart dysfunction** (RV-D) is defined similarly to RV-F, but with a maintained RV-SV. The vast majority of patients with clinical signs of global (biventricular) failure but dominated by failure of the RV or isolated RV-F are 'only' suffering from **right ventricular dysfunction** [3]:

$$\text{RVEDV} \uparrow - \uparrow\uparrow\uparrow \text{ and at the same time } \downarrow - \downarrow\downarrow\downarrow \text{ RV- EF, \textbf{but normal RV-SV}}$$

**Pulmonary hypertension** (PH) must be present when diagnosing RV-D/RV-F [4]. This can be diagnosed when the mean pulmonary pressure > 25 (> 20 [5]) mm Hg at rest [6–9], or > 30 mm Hg with exercise [10] or the systolic pulmonary pressure > 35 mm Hg [6–9] but, of course, LV-dysfunction/failure has to be excluded with a PCWP ≤ 15 mm Hg [9].

Vieillard-Baron [11] defines **RV-D** using echocardiographic evidence of **RV-dilatation** as well as a **leftward shift of the intraventricular septum**.

**Acute cor pulmonale** defines a clinical condition where the **RV is suddenly afterloaded** [12].

## 4.2    Epidemiology and aetiology

Right heart dysfunction/failure has a quite remarkable incidence, affecting approximately 5% of the US population [13] with the outcome largely depending on the underlying cause [14].

Acute RV-D/RV-F due to acute pulmonary hypertension is a common condition in the ITU setting [overview by 2, 12, 15–19]. Most common causes include pulmonary embolism [12], acute respiratory failure [18] (especially in broncho-pulmonary diseases with hypoxic/hypercapnic pulmonary vasoconstriction [19–21] and ARDS [22, 23]), sepsis [14], acutely exacerbated chronic (left/biventricular) heart failure [24, 25] and acute inferior myocardial infarction involving the RV (RV-AMI) [26–28]. Pulmonary vascular resistance (PVR) may be elevated by an increase in lung volume (emphysema) and by a decrease in functional residual capacity, and so lead to RV-D/F [29]. A variety of less common causes includes traumatic injury, fibrosis of the intima of the pulmonary vessels in pulmonary fibrosis, and primary pulmonary hypertension.

Mechanical ventilation (positive pressure ventilation) compromises the pulmonary (micro) circulation through an increase in transpulmonary pressure causing an increase in the systolic load of the RV (↑ RV-afterload) [17, 18, 30–33]. With progressively **increasing tidal volumes** the RV has to generate a higher and higher pressure to open the pulmonary valve and eject blood into the pulmonary vasculature [30, 34]. **PEEP** induces a rise in the intrathoracic pressure [35–39] and, at the very least, higher levels of PEEP (> 8–10 cm $H_2O$) will substantially increase the RV-afterload [35, 40–42].

**RV-F is evoked by an ↑ in PVR and hence by an ↑ RV-afterload** [18].

Failure of the right ventricle is often the final and crucial point in acute critical illness [14, 17, 43]. This is not least because acute right heart failure substantially influences the LV performance in these conditions [44, 45]. In cases where cardiopulmonary resuscitation is necessary patients with moderate or severe pulmonary hypertension are unlikely to survive [46].

## 4.3 Physiological and pathophysiological aspects

## a) General physiology

Previously, very little importance was attached to the right ventricle in the maintenance of the circulation. Laver [44] and his coworkers were the first to show that an acute increase in the resistance of the pulmonary circulation (e.g. resulting from pulmonary embolism) will cause the right ventricle to become the limiting factor of heart function and heart performance [44], due to the acute rise in RV-afterload [18, 47, 48].

The primary functions of the right ventricle comprise [14]:

- maintaining low RA-pressure,
- optimising venous return and
- providing sustained low pressure in the pulmonary vascular bed.

The RV exhibits a sustained ejection during pressure generation and pressure decline with a prolonged low pressure emptying, thus making the ventricle very sensitive to changes in afterload [49]. The RV is responsible for delivering an adequate LV-preload [50, 51].

Acute respiratory failure per se leads to an increase in pulmonary vascular resistance [52] and to a change in pulmonary compliance inducing an increase in RV-afterload [53]. Hypoventilation of the alveoli, hypoxia and/or hypercapnia from respiratory insufficiency (type I and type II) causes an increase in pulmonary pressure and thus promotes PH [4, 6, 54, 55]. ARDS is frequently associated with PH due to an increase in pulmonary vascular resistance (PVR) [52]. PVR is calculated by the ratio of the transpulmonary pressure to the transpulmonary flow [56]:

$$PVR = PAP_{mean} / SV \times HR \; (SV \times HR = CO)$$

Factors contributing to an increase in pulmonary vascular resistance are [57, 58]:

- lung parenchymal destruction,
- airway collapse,
- microthrombi in the pulmonary vessels,
- excessive pulmonary vasoconstriction,
- hypercapnia,
- general and local release of pulmonary vasoconstricting mediators.

It is established that acute respiratory failure leads to an increase in pulmonary vascular resistance, an increase in RV-afterload and reduced RV-function [59–62]. The underlying cellular and molecular pathways are characterized by an imbalance between endogenous vasoconstrictors (in particular endothelin-1) and vasodilators (in particular nitric oxide and prostaglandins) produced and secreted by the pulmonary endothelium leading to an increase in pulmonary vascular resistance and an elevated RV outflow impedance [63–67].

Haemostatic imbalances, probably secondary to pulmonary endothelial dysfunction and/or injury contribute to the rise in PVR [10].

An increased PVR (which accompanies PH) leads to an increase in RVEDV and a decrease in RV-EF and thus, at the very least, to RV-dysfunction [68]. Furthermore, high pulmonary pressure (PH) exerts an increased load on RV ejection, thus inducing an increase in the RV-afterload [47, 69, 70].

The right heart is very poorly adapted to conditions of raised afterload [71] and a normal RV is not able to acutely increase the mean PA pressure above 40 mm Hg [72]; hence, rapid haemodynamic compromise and an early onset of hypotension and shock will occur in patients with predominant RV-F [71]. The RV and RA typically (immediately [16, 22]) dilate in response to acute right heart volume [73, 74] or pressure loading [16, 22, 73, 75, 76].

Normally crescent shaped in cross-section with a concave free wall and a convex septum [77], the RV has a markedly lower volume to surface ratio in comparison to the LV and thus a much greater compliance [78]. These features of the RV predispose to significant RV-dilatation if afterload increases acutely [78]. The dilatation enables the RV to maintain SV [16, 22] (utilisation of preload reserve [79] via the Frank-Starling mechanism [72]) fulfilling the criteria for RV-dysfunction [12, 16, 17, 76]. Recently, Kerbaul has shown that a reduction in RV contractility may occur as well [69, 70].

(Sudden) ↑ in pressure (volume) load of the RV causing PH [15–19, 57, 58]                →
↑ **RV-afterload/RV outflow impedance** [12, 16, 17, 69, 75, 76]
↓

- **RV-dilatation** (↑ **RVEDV/RVEDD**) [12, 16, 17, 75, 76, 78] (acute and rapid / or extensive volume loading, in particular over a certain limit [80] primarily causes RV-dilatation [73, 74]),
- ↓ **RV-EF** [12, 16, 17, 76, 81],
- ↓ **RV contractility** [47, 69, 70],
- ↑ **Heart Rate** (often the first attempt to compensate acute RV pressure and/or volume load [17, 82])
↓

**Right heart dysfunction** [68, 81] (**RV-SV maintained in the first instance** [81]).

Furthermore, in case of a sudden rise in RV-afterload / increase in RV-outflow impedance and/or a loss in contractility [83, 84] the resulting RV dilatation [11, 12, 16, 76, 78, 82] and the fall in RV-EF [11, 12, 16, 76] are accompanied by a marked rise in RVEDP [75, 85–88]. This implies a rise in pericardial pressure (PP) [88–97] since RA pressure reflects the RVEDP [91, 92, 96, 97] and correlates well to PP under physiological [98–100] as well as in pathological conditions [94, 95, 98]. Therefore in RV-D with concomitant increase in RVEDP the PP will rise as well [88, 89, 91–93, 95].

Right heart dysfunction → ↑ RVEDP and thus ↑ PP

[12, 16, 17, 75, 76, 85–88, 90–95, 98–100].

The pericardial pressure exerted on the right and left ventricle are similar in most conditions, with the exception of circumstances where the afterload is increased considerably to one ventricle alone [101–103], e.g. acute and chronic pulmonary hypertension [104–106]. RV-D/RV-F always implies an increase in PP [102] and, due to diastolic ventricular interaction (DVI), changes in filling pressure are more pronounced on the RV than on the LV [24, 25, 101, 107].

## b)      Diastolic ventricular interactions

The global hemodynamic consequences of RV-D are dependent on the critical **interaction between the two ventricles** [108, 109]. Under physiological conditions we will find similar end-diastolic volumes in RV and LV [12, 110, 111]. The heart chambers are enclosed by the pericardium and share the interventricular septum and, as such, **ventricular interactions** occur [25, 112–115]. This interaction mainly occurs in diastole (therefore named diastolic ventricular interaction, **DVI**) and changes (particularly **sudden** changes [25, 101, 112, 113, 115]) in the end-diastolic volume (and intraventricular pressure) of one ventricle will directly influence the volume (and intraventricular pressure and thus compliance [115]) of the other ventricle [25, 101, 116, 117].

These diastolic interactions are mediated via the shared structures of the ventricles, the interventricular septum and the pericardium with its constraining effects on ventricular filling through poor distensibility [88, 118, 119]. Thus, an increase in the cross-sectional area of one ventricle, i.e. due to volume loading or enlargement, necessarily reduces the area of the opposite ventricle (resulting in less filling volume), simultaneously causing an increase in the pericardial pressure (PP) [24, 88]. The total cardiac volume (filling) remains unchanged [88, 89]. Therefore the pericardium plays a key role in the loading conditions [113, 120, 121] and this is particularly seen in the acute situation.

The increase in RVEDV which, accompanied by a rise in RVEDP and PP, shifts the interventricular septum towards the LV cavity during diastole. This occurs subject to the restrictions imposed by the acutely non distensible pericardium on the RV as the RV-cavity size increases [14, 122].

Furthermore, Kingma showed that in acute RV pressure or volume load the interventricular septum becomes flattened or even concave at end-diastole due to RV dilatation and raised RVEDP, diminishing the trans-septal pressure gradient (trans-septal pressure gradient = LVEDP – RVEDP [123]) and pushing the septum towards the left ventricle [123]. Numerous publications confirm the change in the septum position in different conditions such as acute and chronic pulmonary hypertension [101, 104, 107, 124], congestive heart failure [24, 25] and mechanical ventilation [125]. The leftward shift of the septum and the constraining effects of the pericardium compress the LV with a resultant decrease in LV-size and in end-diastolic LV-filling (reduced LVEDV) [14, 122, 126], producing a reduction in LV-SV [127, 128]. Furthermore, the LV diastolic properties are affected as well, and the reduction in LV compliance in so far contributes to the compromised LV-filling and, hence, the reduction in LV-SV [14, 73, 122, 134]: This is due to the flattening of the septum as RV dilates and as the RVEDP rises, LV compliance will be reduced [14, 73, 133], resulting in altered LV diastolic function (dysfunction) with abnormal LV relaxation and reduced LV compliance (LV diastolic dysfunction) [14, 73, 122, 133].

$\uparrow$ RV-afterload $\rightarrow \uparrow$ RVEDD/RVEDV $\rightarrow \rightarrow \downarrow$ LVEDD/LVEDV $\quad \rightarrow \downarrow$ LV-SV

[73,75,105,113,129–132]

LV-compliance $\downarrow$ [14, 72, 73, 122, 133]  $\quad \rightarrow \downarrow$ LV-SV

## c)      The role of the pericardium in diastolic-ventricular interaction

The constraining effect of the pericardium not only reduces and limits the LV-filling but also the dilatation and filling of the RV as well. Under normal conditions RVEDP and PP are low, but in cases of raised intra-thoracic pressure [135], elevated external pressure is exerted on the heart [35, 93, 136, 137], exhibiting a constraining effect particularly on the thin walled RV [101, 124]. Both RVEDP and LVEDP will rise, but the rise affects the RVEDP (and hence PP) more than the LVEDP ($\uparrow$ RVEDP > $\uparrow$ LVEDP) [35, 101, 124]. In regard to DVI, changes in filling pressure are more pronounced in the RV than in the LV and thus volume loading would increase RVEDP more than LVEDP, whilst unloading, the fall in RVEDP exceeds the fall in LVEDP [24, 25, 101, 107]. **Right-sided HF** always implies an increased PP [102] and thus constraint should always be considered.

Ventricular interaction due to pericardial constraint is diminished as long as the PP is < 5 mm Hg [138]. In the thin walled RV, if RVEDP $\geq$ 4 mm Hg, PP will increase in a parallel fashion [139]. A PP exceeding 9–10 mm Hg will exert substantial constraint on ventricular filling [93, 139]. When LVEDP exceeds 10–15 mm Hg, the LVEDP-LVEDV relation becomes much steeper and the pericardium limits further increases in LV end-diastolic volume [140, 141].

As discussed in chapter 1, the CVP reflects the pericardial pressure [95, 98], and pericardial constraint accounts for 96% of the RA pressure, if CVP > 10 mm Hg [93].

The ability to maintain an adequate RV-SV by RV-dilatation is very limited. RV-SV decreases almost linearly with an abrupt increase in afterload as soon as pulmonary hypertension (PAP > 25 mm Hg) occurs, despite all compensatory attempts (RV-dilatation) [142]. Very soon the constraint exerted by the pericardium will restrict the dilatation and further fluid administration in order to increase RVEDV and thus ensure a proper RV-SV is, if at all, only of marginal help. Contrary to previous belief, fluid administration will be harmful because any further dilation of the RV cannot correct an LV-filling deficit and may reduce LV-filling even more [45, 87, 101, 116, 124, 143–145]. If **RV-D occurs**, no further fluid administration is advisable, volume loading will be **harmful** [145–147] in the failing RV, volume **unloading** will **increase** the SV/CO [146, 147].

Furthermore, compensated RV-D/RV-F quickly deteriorates (to end-stage) [14] through a vicious cycle of **auto-aggravation** which is unique to the RV [14].

## d)      Auto-aggravation

**RV-dilatation** (RVEDV $\uparrow$) **and the alteration of the RV-geometry** secondary to the increased RV-afterload or substantial volume loading leads to a **tricuspid annulus dilatation and func-**

tional tricuspid insufficiency (TR) [79, 148, 149] which is further aggravated by the increased RVEDP [14, 79]. The tricuspid regurgitation leads to congestion in the hepatic and renal vascular bed and to a fall in RV-SV [14, 79] which is, as per definition, RV-F. Less blood volume will be ejected into the pulmonary vasculature due to the fact that the PA-pressure is higher than that on the venous side and, due to the TR, ejection into the low pressure conduit is easier. The reduced RV-SV implies a further (additional to the reduction of LV filling secondary to the DVI effect) reduction in LV preload via the so called series effect [106, 150].

## e)    Series effect

The two ventricles are coupled in a row (series), one after the other, and thus the output necessarily is equal over time [51, 116]. Therefore, a reduction in right ventricular output results in less blood (volume) being transported to the LV [106, 150]. Less filling of the LV (less LV-preload) will result in a (further) fall in LV-SV as per the Frank-Starling mechanism [127, 128].

'The performance of the RV determines LV-preload' [51].

Due to systemic vasoconstriction the systemic arterial BP is usually maintained in the initial phase [151]; however, with a further and now substantial decrease in LV preload causing considerable loss of LV-SV, a BP drop is inevitable [79, 152, 153]. RV-F is often accompanied by hypotension [108, 154]. Kerbaul [69, 70] and Bellamy [155] showed that, unfortunately in this situation, we cannot expect an increase in contractility to maintain or increase the RV-SV.

The combination of autoaggravation and the series effect can be summarized below:

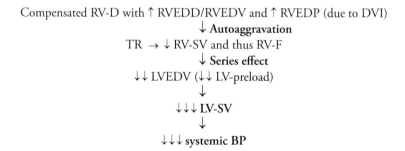

Compensated RV-D with ↑ RVEDD/RVEDV and ↑ RVEDP (due to DVI)
↓ Autoaggravation
TR → ↓ RV-SV and thus RV-F
↓ Series effect
↓↓ LVEDV (↓↓ LV-preload)
↓
↓↓↓ LV-SV
↓
↓↓↓ systemic BP

[1, 2, 3, 14, 79, 106, 108, 127, 128, 150, 152–154].

## f)    Pulmonary hypertension and ischaemia

An elevated PA-pressure puts the RV at risk of myocardial ischaemia [18, 47, 48], with or without pre-existing coronary artery disease [156, 157] and RV-F may occur as a result of the ischaemia [158]. RV-dilatation increases the likelihood that ischaemia will develop because, at a certain point, a critical increase in wall tension and stress (secondary to RV enlargement) occurs, producing a significant mismatch between oxygen supply and demand [79].

With an increase in RV-afterload, the isovolumetric contraction phase and ejection time are prolonged and an increase in RV myocardial oxygen consumption results [14, 76, 159]. An increased oxygen demand would normally be compensated by a substantial increase in RCA-perfusion [159, 160] but, in cases of low RCA perfusion, there is a high risk that RV myocardial ischaemia will further worsen the RV-function [87, 108, 152, 159, 160]. As RV-F is often accompanied by hypotension predominantly secondary to the reduction in LV-SV as described above – resulting in a marked reduction in myocardial perfusion [154, 158, 159, 161] – the worst case scenario occurs, the **combination of PH and ischaemia** [87, 152, 159, 162].

The development of an **ischaemic right ventricular myocardium** [2, 18, 87, 152, 158, 161] may be the **final step in the pathophysiological cascade of RV-F** and means that life threatening heart failure will almost inevitably develop [2, 87, 152, 162].

Ischaemia of the right ventricular myocardium occurs when RCA-perfusion pressure < 25–30 mm Hg [158, 161]; in the case of PH, the RCA-perfusion pressure has to be > 45 mm Hg in order to avoid ischaemia [161] and, if a significant RCA stenosis is present, an even higher perfusion pressure is required [2, 158, 163].

**RV-afterload and ischaemia are the decisive factors determining the pathophysiology of RV-D/RV-F [2, 18, 47, 87, 108, 152, 158, 159, 162].**

## g)    The interventricular septum and the apex

In critical situations such as acute RV pressure or volume load, and particularly when RV ischaemia develops, the interventricular septum (IVS) 'behaves' as a **functional part of the RV** [164, 165]. Under acute RV pressure or volume load the IVS during systole moves towards the RV in a 'paradoxical' fashion. This 'paradoxical' septal movement is an active process of the interventricular septum at the end of systole allowing prolongation of the RV contraction phase, whilst the LV starts to relax [12], moving towards the RV-cavity and increasing the RV contractile force [12, 144, 166]. The loss of the contractility of the septum under such conditions will markedly worsen the haemodynamic situation [108], but inotropic drugs in this situation may augment the RV systolic function by improving the contractility of the IVS [165, 167, 168].

Furthermore, the contraction of the apex of the heart contributes in cases of RV-D/RV-F to the net contractility of the right ventricle as well [165, 169].

Therefore if either the septum or apex fails, e.g., myocardial infarction, the decrease in LV contractility may result in RV-F [170].

The functional behaviour described above is in accordance with the anatomy. The shared pericardium and septum, the mutually encircling epicardial fibres, and the attachment of the RV free wall to the anterior and posterior parts of the septum allow the apex and the septum to make a contribution to systolic RV function [67].

## h)    The left ventricle

As described, the left and right ventricles are inter-related. LV dysfunction/failure affects RV-function, leading to RV-D/RV-F in several ways. LV-dysfunction may increase the RV-afterload due to pulmonary congestion [67], and/or because of a reduced MAP, the RCA perfusion may decrease, leading to RV-ischaemia [171]. However, LV-dysfunction also exerts an influence on lung mechanics and gas exchange [172], with a reduction in lung volume and lung compliance [173, 174].

# i)   Mechanical ventilation

Mechanical (positive pressure) ventilation [18, 30, 32, 33, 175, 176] and the application of PEEP [36–39, 53, 177] increase the intrathoracic pressure (pleural pressure). Artucio [178] and Brienza [179] demonstrated that the application of PEEP and/or positive pressure ventilation may lead to a rise in transpulmonary pressure and an increase in RV-outflow impedance [30–33]. Increasing tidal volumes raise intrathoracic pressure [30, 34] resulting in a marked elevation of the transpulmonary pressure with the potential risk to cause an acute cor pulmonale as found in a substantial number of patients [180]. Transpulmonary pressure directly correlates with RV-afterload [34] and since transpulmonary pressure rises in positive pressure ventilation and PEEP use, RV-outflow impedance will increase [35, 174, 181], which may promote the development of RV-D.

RV-function may also be compromised via another mechanism:
With increasing pleural (intrathoracic) pressure, we find an impairment of LV- and RV-compliance: RV-compliance decreases markedly with only small increases in pleural pressure whilst the LV-compliance decreases with a significant amount only with higher increases in pleural pressure [35, 40]. As a consequence, the steep rise in RVEDP associated with only very small increases in RV end-diastolic filling [35] is accompanied by a parallel rise in PP with the potential to cause DVI (see chapter 1.8 and DVI of this chapter).

Pleural pressure is directly transmitted to the pericardial space [182] and so an increase in pleural pressure will increase the PP. Therefore, the normally low RVEDP and PP will rise markedly in mechanical ventilation, pneumonia, ARDS, etc and so will contribute to an ↑ in the pressure surrounding the heart [94]. Any rise in pleural pressure will, via a concomitant rise in PP, limit the distending capacity of the cardiac cavities and will exert a constraining effect on both RV and, to a lesser extent, on the LV [40].

Furthermore, with mechanical ventilation the venous return is compromised, reducing the RV-filling and function and will hence reduce the RV-SV [183].

However, positive pressure ventilation and PEEP are not always detrimental. There is evidence that relatively low PEEP levels ($\leq 8$–10 cm $H_2O$) have beneficial effects on the pulmonary haemodynamics and do not increase the RV-afterload significantly, even though the pleural pressure and thus the transpulmonary pressure are elevated [41]. Schmitt [184] found that the use of a low PEEP improved the blood flow through the pulmonary vessel bed, reducing the RV-afterload and the risk of RV-D. The reasons behind these beneficial effects are:

- Air (gas) trapping is often present in respiratory failure due to chest infection or ARDS and increases the pleural pressure, the trans-pulmonary pressure, and the pulmonary vascular resistance. Gas trapping is relieved by (low) PEEP, hence reducing transpulmonary pressure and improving blood flow through a reduction in pulmonary vascular resistance [40, 185];
- (Low) PEEP is beneficial in diseased and stiff lungs/lung compartments as it improves blood

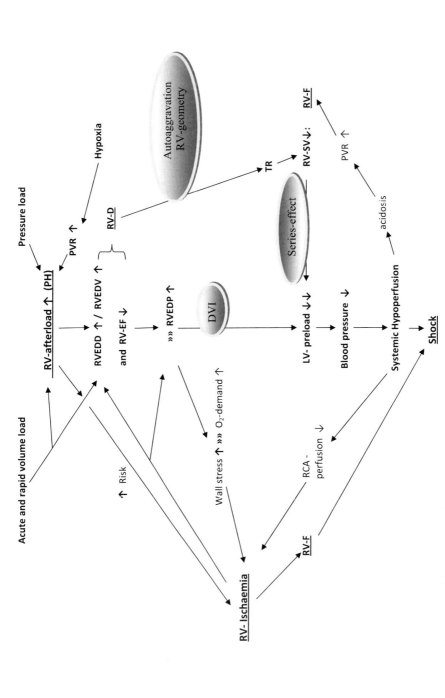

**Figure 4.1** Pathophysiology of right heart dysfunction and failure. Literature to this diagram which is developed by the authors: See physiological and pathophysiological aspects, and Taichman, SCCM 34th congress 15–19th Jan 2005, as well as Kucher, N  Acute Cardiac Care Meeting of the ESC, Prague Oct 23rd 2006.

flow in the pulmonary vascular bed [40, 184–186]. Interestingly the PEEP-levels mentioned above, which are beneficial for pulmonary haemodynamics, correspond to those called 'best PEEP' described by Sutter in 1975 [186]. He found PEEP levels around $8 \pm 4$ cm $H_2O$ resulted in optimal oxygenation transport in ARDS patients. So, these PEEP levels seem to be beneficial for both the treatment of the respiratory failure and the maintenance of a sufficient cardiac function. There is no doubt, however, that PEEP levels > 10–12 cm $H_2O$ exert a significant RV pressure load (increased RV-afterload) and cause a leftward shift of the interventricular septum, producing RV-D [40];

- PEEP will decrease LV-afterload which will, in the situation of LV-failure through mechanisms described previously, have a beneficial effect on RV function [187–189]:

$$PEEP \rightarrow \uparrow \text{intrathoracic pressure} \rightarrow \text{transmural LVEDP} \downarrow \rightarrow \text{LV wall stress} \downarrow \rightarrow$$
$$\text{LV afterload} \downarrow [40, 176, 190].$$

However, it has to be stressed that, in case of pre-existing and/or manifest RV-D/RV-F, PEEP was found to increase RV-afterload in every case and may worsen the hemodynamic situation by its net effect [191].

## 4.4    Diagnostic aspects

### a)    Clinical features

There are a lack of specific **clinical signs** in acute right heart dysfunction or failure [160] but, nevertheless, the following suggestive signs may be present [14, 17]:

- Neck vein distension
- Positive hepato-jugular reflex
- Renal impairment with oligo-anuria
- Tachypnoea is present in up to 80% [192]
- Hepato-/hepato-splenomegaly
- Abdominal discomfort
- Hypotension
- Peripheral oedema*
- evated lactate, disturbed coagulation and raised liver enzymes may by an expression of liver dysfunction due to hepatic congestion [160].

*Peripheral oedema is not unique to RV-D/RV-F, it is secondary to hyperaldosteronism induced by hypercapnic acidosis, hypoxaemia and renal insufficiency [193, 194], and chronic venous insufficiency.

### b)    Serum biomarkers

**BNP** has a strong, positive correlation to PVR and RVEDP in patients suffering from primary pulmonary hypertension [195, 196]. BNP rises gradually with increasing severity of RV-D/RV-F [197–199]. However, the thresholds of when to diagnose RV-D (RV-F) are still in discussion and vary from between > 50 pg/ml [200] and > 100 pg/ml [201]. Furthermore, elevated BNP levels may be present in chronic RV-D and chronic PH [196, 202, 203].

Troponin I > 0.1 µg/l (pathologically elevated) was found **only** in severe RV-D caused by pulmonary embolism [200]. Its occurrence is associated with early mortality [204, 205]. In the case of pulmonary embolism, patients with a negative serum troponin and normal ECG are at the lowest risk [206].

Both, Troponin and BNP have excellent negative predictive value and tend to exclude a complicated hospital stay when negative on admission [207, 208].

## c)      Electrocardiography

**ECG ST-elevation** (> 0.1 mV) in $V_{R3}$ and/or $V_{R4}$ in patients with **inferior ST-elevation acute myocardial infarction** is highly specific for RV-ischaemia due to a proximal RCA-lesion (sensitivity 83%, specificity 77%) [28, 43]. Involvement of the RV, as a complication of acute inferior myocardial infarction (ST-elevation in II, III, aVF [209]) is to be expected in approximately 50% [26].

## d)      Echocardiography

Direct pressure and volume measurements can be made using a **Swan-Ganz-conductance catheter** [210] and right heart catheterisation was previously the method of choice, but due to favourable comparisons to **echocardiography**, the latter, less invasive method is now widely used [211], and an echocardiographic assessment is **essential in establishing the diagnosis of RV-D/RV-F** [12, 17, 201, 212–215]. Vieillard-Baron [11] requires only the finding of **RV-dilatation with a leftward shift of the septum** in order to make a **diagnosis of RV-D**; however, there are many other echocardiographic features of RV-D/RV-F which can be used to confirm the diagnosis:

- The RV is clearly dilated when the RV size ≥ LV size [17, 192, 212, 213, 216]. The most common criteria with which to diagnose RV-dilatation is the RV/LV-ratio (assessed in the four-chamber view), but there is disagreement about the thresholds indicative of significant RV-dilatation, ranging from a ratio of 0.6 to 1.0 [217–219];
- The IVS becomes flat and bows towards the left ventricle in end-diastole; the right ventricle becomes circular at end-diastole while the LV becomes eccentric in shape [12, 212, 213] with a dyskinetic/paradoxical IVS movement, which is due to systolic RV overload [201]. **Paradoxical septal movement** is generally a sign of an **acute increase in RV-afterload** [220];
- The tricuspid annular plane systolic excursion (**TAPSE**) is an easy to use and very valuable parameter in assessing right heart function [221, 222]. It is merely the AV-displacement of the tricuspid valve.
  TAPSE shows a good inverse correlation to the pulmonary vascular resistance (TAPSE ~ 1/PVR) representing pulmonary hypertension in cases of elevated resistance [221]. **TAPSE is afterload dependent** and **pathological values indicate an elevated RV-afterload** [221]. It is an excellent measure of the systolic RV-function [223–225] as it has a direct correlation with RV-EF (**TAPSE ~ RV-EF**) [222, 224, 226, 227]. TAPSE is a highly sensitive and specific parameter of depressed RV-SV [228] as RV-SV indirectly correlates with PVR [229].

Additionally, a good indirect correlation is established between the severity of the tricuspid regurgitation (TR) and TAPSE (TAPSE ~ 1/ TR) [221]. A normal TAPSE value is > 22 mm [221, 230–232], 15–19 mm excursion indicates a moderate depression of TAPSE [221] and if < 15 mm the outcome is very poor [221]. However, **TAPSE < 18 mm** indicates a RV-LV disproportion reflecting the **series** and **interdependent** (DVI) **effects** of the **failing RV on the LV-filling** [233];

- Hypokinesis of the free RV wall [201];
- A TR-jet velocity of > 2.7 m/s is suggestive of pulmonary hypertension [201];
- Inferior vena-cava diameter (sub-costal view) > 10 mm during inspiration (in spontaneously breathing patients) provides evidence for pathology [201]; if the amount of collapse is < 50%, a pathologically high pressure is present, indicating pressure and/or volume (over)load [234]. In mechanically ventilated patients the venous flow to the right heart is markedly reduced during inspiration secondary to the positive intrathoracic pressure reducing the amount of vena cava and hepatic vein collapse [235];
- If of special interest, the pulmonary vascular resistance (PVR) may be calculated using echocardiographic parameters. PVR is calculated by the ratio of transpulmonary pressure ($\Delta p$) to transpulmonary flow (Qp):

$$PVR = \Delta p / Qp;$$

- TR (maximal tricuspid regurgitant velocity) and $TVI_{RVOT}$ (time-velocity interval of the right ventricular outflow tract) can be used as a correlate to $\Delta p$ (TR) and Qp ($TVI_{RVOT}$) [236, 237]:

$$PVR = TR/TVI_{RVOT.}$$

Due to the Bernoulli equation, TR will increase as systolic PA pressure increases [236, 238, 239];

- Abbas [240] found a very good correlation between $PVR_{cath}$ (measured invasively) and $TR/TVI_{RVOT}$ with a correlation coefficient r = 0.93, CI 0.87–0.96:

**$TR/TVI_{RVOT}$ < 0.2 is most likely to be normal with PVR < 150 dyn × s × cm$^{-5}$**
(80 dyn × s × cm$^{-5}$ equals one Wood unit [241]):

- **The combination of a small and well contracting LV and a big, dilated and poorly contract-ing RV is pathognomonic for 'acute' right heart failure** [242];
- Interestingly, McConnell [220] has described severe hypokinesia of the mid free wall of the RV, but with a normally contracting apex, as pathognomonic of pulmonary embolism.

Features indicating possible **de-compensation** of RV-F are [67]:
- Rising RVEDP,
- worsening diastolic RV-dysfunction [243] (becoming obvious by an inadequate increase in RVEDP),
- ↓ LV-SV and markedly LV diastolic dysfunction (induced by an ↑ in RV-size and ↑ RVEDP [80, 244]).

## 4.5    Therapy

It has been emphasised that RV-afterload (PH) and ischaemia are the decisive factors in precipitating RV-D/RV-F and the ability to therapeutically ameliorate these factors will determine the prognosis [2, 18, 47, 87, 108, 152, 158, 245]. Thus, reduction of the elevated RV-afterload and avoidance or reversal of RCA-hypoperfusion are the essential issues which therapy must address [47, 108, 246–251]:

- **Critical reduction of the increased RV-afterload**
- **Avoidance/treatment of right ventricular myocardial ischaemia**

Acute RV-F/acute exacerbation of RV-D/RV-F are reversible if the cause of the increased afterload can be treated [14, 18].

Additional targets are:
- Treatment of underlying disease [14, 17, 18]
- Improvement of RV contractility to overcome critical acute situations [44, 70, 249, 252]

Remember, the hemodynamic consequences of RV-D/RV-F are the result of a critical interaction between both ventricles [108, 109].

## a)        **Specific measures** [overview by 14, 17, 18]:

- Thrombolytic therapy/PCI in case of acute coronary syndrome [253–257]
- Thrombolytic therapy/catheter fractioning or embolectomy in pulmonary embolism
- Specific treatment of broncho-pulmonary disease
- Treatment of systemic sepsis
- ARDS: Therapy of underlying disease
- Correction of valvular heart disease, and left heart failure

In acute myocardial infarction with involvement of the RV early reperfusion by thrombolysis or primary PCI is essential [253–257].

**Right heart dysfunction/failure and pulmonary embolism:**
RV-F is the most common cause of death within 30 days following PE [258, 259] and RV dysfunction is known to cause an increased mortality [258, 260–261].
   50% of all patients with pulmonary embolism present as clinically stable, without hypotension or circulatory failure, although suffering from RV-D [201, 258, 263 ]. They are at high risk of haemodynamic instability or even death during the first days after admission [263, 264].
   The Shock Index is a sensitive parameter which can easily be used in daily practice in order to assess the potential outcome of patients with pulmonary embolism [79].

$$\text{Shock Index = HR/sBP} \geq 1 \rightarrow \text{mortality ++}$$

Thus, patients with a positive (≥ 1) shock index should be treated by thrombolysis (Evidence level A, Class I) [265–269].

Although not all studies give convincing evidence about the predictive and prognostic value of RV dysfunction [260, 261], Kucher [262] established that **RV dysfunction is an independent prognostic predictor** by analysing the data of the famous ICOPER study [258]. Patients with a systolic blood pressure ≥ 90 mm Hg (and thus classified as being hemodynamically stable/with preserved BP) but with RV-dysfunction had almost double the risk of death (16.3%) in comparison to those without RV-dysfunction (9.4%) over the first 30 days. Thus, although initially haemodynamically stable, all patients with RV dysfunction are at a high risk of death [262]. These results are consistent with those reported by Figulla [260], who found a 5–8% mortality rate in patients with normal BP but with RV dysfunction, while the prognosis of all patients without RV dysfunction was excellent (mortality rate 0–1%). It should be noted that the level of blood pressure taken as normal (sBP of > 90 mm Hg versus > 120 mm Hg respectively) was different in both studies and that the blood pressure on admission has a substantial impact on the patient's prognosis [260] (see Table 1):

Table 4.1  Impact of blood pressure on patient's prognosis

| Clinical Scenario | Mortality during hospital stay |
| --- | --- |
| Normal BP, without RV-dysfunction | 0–1% |
| Normal BP, with RV-dysfunction | 5–8% |
| Hypotension, without signs of shock | 15% |
| Hypotension and shock | up to 35% |

Not all studies have concluded that thrombolytic therapy reduces the mortality significantly, when administered to clinically stable patients with RV-D but preserved BP [260, 261]. Nevertheless, the haemodynamic situation clearly improved and stabilised immediately after the patients received thrombolytic agents [258, 261, 264, 270–272]. Furthermore, the first prospective study assessing the long term outcome after first-time 'submassive' pulmonary embolism in previously healthy patients treated by heparin and warfarin found 41% of the patients either with persistent or subsequently (weeks to months after PE) developed RV abnormalities or functional limitations [273]. The authors suggest that first-time pulmonary embolism is able to cause persistent right heart damage or to initiate a process which damages the RV over time. The main pathological mechanisms involved appear initially to be ischaemia of the RV subendocardium followed by an inflammatory response [274–276].

The results by Kucher [262], Figulla [260] and Woods [79] suggest that patients in shock and those with hypotension need thrombolytic treatment, but it would also seem more than wise – based on the current evidence – to consider patients with established proof of RV-dysfunction on an individual basis for thrombolysis as well.

## b)  Adjunctive therapy [14, 17, 18, 192, 277]

### i)  Fluid management and optimization of preload
The recommendations regarding fluid management in acute RV-D and RV-F have completely changed in recent years following a large amount of discussion [14, 51, 229, 277, 278]. RV filling above the physiological limit is accompanied by RV-dilatation [279]; thus, in RV-D (and

particularly, of course, in RV-F) fluid administration should be avoided because a beneficial effect of volume expansion cannot be expected, even if there is a low LV-preload [51, 146, 147]. (Further) volume administration in this situation will not increase RV-SV and hence CO; in a depressed RV or in manifest RV-F only **volume unloading** will increase CO [146, 147]. This potentially harmful reaction to volume loading is the result of DVI, aggravation of RV-dilatation accompanied by worsened TR, and ischaemia as described previously in this chapter. Therefore, in the **vast majority of patients suffering from acute RV-D/RV-F volume loading has no benefit** at all [14, 24, 51, 101, 116, 146, 147, 229, 278].

However, there are some exceptions to this rule. In the (few) cases of RV-F with **normal PVR** volume loading may be beneficial and increase preload, leading to an increase in RV-SV and LV-SV [278]. Furthermore, patients suffering from **acute myocardial infarction with significant involvement of the right ventricle** are probably the group who will **benefit most from controlled and balanced volume loading** [108].

Ideally in daily practice, an echocardiogram to clarify the diagnosis, to assess the hemodynamic situation, and to guide therapy should be performed as soon as RV-D/RV-F and/or biventricular failure are suspected. However, as an emergency measure in shock or in haemodynamic instability [280–283], as long as no clinical signs of fluid overload are present, a careful and well monitored fluid challenge seems to be appropriate [280–282, 284, 285].

### ii)      Vasopressors: treatment and avoidance of ischaemia

Vasopressors directly increase the systemic blood pressure and thus improve the perfusion pressure of the RCA [158, 286–289]. Ghignone and others [245, 290] were first to establish that vasopressors may be the critical element in the treatment of acute right heart failure, as the administration of vasopressor drugs can break the pathological vicious cycle and avoid the manifestation of RV myocardial ischaemia [2, 87, 152, 245, 290].

Agents that increase the aortic pressure are able to reverse RV ischaemia and actually improve RV function. Vlahakes [158] demonstrated that an increase in RCA coronary perfusion pressure will directly increase the net perfusion of the myocardium, certainly for the right ventricle [158, 291] and probably for the LV myocardium as well [291]. As mentioned in Chapter 2, *Noradrenaline* is the vasopressor of choice, as it is in hypotensive, life-threatening situations where vasopressor administration is essential [249, 286–289, 292–296], not only restoring arterial pressure but improving RV-contractility as well [108, 154].

For practical purposes, the coronary perfusion pressure (CPP) is determined for the left ventricle by the equation [297]:

$$\text{CPP = diastolic blood pressure – LVEDP}$$

The right ventricle under physiological conditions is perfused continuously throughout systole and diastole. In PH the CPP depends on the difference between diastolic blood pressure and RVEDP [160]:

$$\text{CPP = diastolic blood pressure – RVEDP, or}$$
$$\text{CPP = diastolic blood pressure – CVP}$$

Ischaemia is known to occur in healthy persons if the CCP in the RCA is as low as ≤ 25–30 mm Hg [158, 161]. In PH, a CCP > 45 mm Hg is necessary to avoid ischaemia [161], but generally a CPP > 50 mm Hg is essential in order to provide basic perfusion of the myocardium [298, 299], and coronary autoregulation functions from approximately 60 mm Hg to 140 mm Hg [300, 301]. This means that in PH, and if the CVP > 10 mm Hg, a *diastolic blood pressure* > 55–60 mm Hg is required and, in order to maintain coronary artery autoregulation, a MAP > 65–70 mm Hg is essential.

### iii)     Critical RV-afterload reduction

The **reduction** of the pulmonary vascular resistance (**RV-afterload**) is, alongside avoidance and reversal of ischaemia, the **central aim of therapy** in patients suffering from pulmonary hypertension and RV-dysfunction/failure [47, 108, 246–249]. A reduction in RV-afterload will reduce RV $O_2$ consumption and will reverse the pathophysiological processes described, breaking the vicious cycle [14].

*Treatment of underlying disease and reducing pulmonary hypertension*
In patients suffering from acute exacerbations of COPD a **combination of β-agonist agents and anticholinergic agents** (bronchodilator therapy), preferably nebulised, is standard therapy in order to reduce airway resistance and vasoconstriction of pulmonary vessels (as well as v-a-shunts) [302–304].

In patients with COPD, methylxanthines (e.g. aminophylline) are effective in reducing the pulmonary vascular resistance, increasing RV-EF and RV-contractility [305, 306]. However, they are not recommended to be routinely added to the bronchodilator therapy [303, 304, 307, 308] (and some regard them obsolete [229]) due to the frequent and often severe side-effects potentially causing deterioration of the overall cardiac function, malignant rhythm disturbances, worsening a-v-shunting (producing a further reduction in arterial oxygen content) and tachycardia increasing $O_2$ consumption, risking ventricular ischaemia and exacerbating the final step in the vicious cycle [307, 308]. They should only be considered in patients with an exacerbation of COPD [307, 308] who have RV-F resistant to all other therapeutic measures and where it seems reasonable to continue in patients who were taking them prior to the exacerbation [303].

In severe asthma, magnesium has a synergistic beneficial effect with $β_2$-agonists and should be considered [309].

*Symptomatic treatment of PH: Vasodilators*
**Systemic vasodilators** are highly unselective and, unfortunately, will worsen the ventilation-perfusion mismatch resulting in reduced arterial oxygen saturation, as well as reducing RCA perfusion (by lowering the systemic blood pressure) resulting in or worsening RV myocardial ischaemia [310, 311]. Thus, although vasodilators such as GTN or nitroprusside may reduce the resistance of the pulmonary vasculature [14, 17], they should normally only play an adjunctive role in therapy, but may be considered in normotensive patients who are fluid overloaded [2].

**Inhaled pulmonary vasodilators exert highly specific and local effects**: Prostaglandins (e.g. Iloprost, a synthetic prostaglandin $I_2$) and their analogues such as nitric oxide (NO) show vasodilating effects selectively on the pulmonary vasculature [312–315], thus NO and Iloprost are very effective in reducing PVR [316]. Nebulised prostaglandins exert beneficial effects in patients with primarily pulmonary hypertension (PPH) and acute right heart failure [317] as well as other situations with secondary pulmonary hypertension and acute RV-failure [318–320]. No significant toxic effects of prostaglandins are known and they lower the pulmonary arterial pressure more effectively than NO [321, 322]. Unfortunately a concomitant reduction of mortality rate when administered in acute cases has not yet been established [320]. In desperate, life-threatening situations prostaglandins should be considered, although they are currently not licensed in Europe for cases of acute RV-failure due to secondary pulmonary hypertension [17].

Inhalation of NO will only reach and cause vasodilatation in ventilated areas. The reflex hypoxic pulmonary vasoconstriction (Euler-Liljestrand reflex) will act and thus an increase in v-a shunt volume will be avoided [323]. Administration of NO improves RV-pump function and reduces RV-dilatation in patients with COPD and ARDS [23]. Importantly, however, NO exhibits a rebound phenomenon after stopping the administration [324]. Although currently only licensed for use in primary pulmonary hypertension (PPH) of the newborn, it may be considered in cases of severe acute RV failure refractory to conservative treatment strategies [12].

**Sildenafil** (a specific phosphodiesterase-5 inhibitor) exerts beneficial acute and chronic haemodynamic effects by lowering the pulmonary pressure in patients with pulmonary hypertension [9, 325–327]. It has been shown to reduce PA pressure and to increase CO alone or in combination with nitric oxide in stable patients [328, 329]. The effect commences soon after administration, with peak haemodynamic effects occurring within one hour and lasting three to four hours. Sildenafil has potential to lower systemic blood pressure, causing hypotension, and so caution is warranted in critically ill patients [330].

### iv)       Improvement of RV systolic function/contractility
As previously described, the IVS [164, 165] and the apex [165, 169] play a direct and significant role in maintaining RV function. The LV contributes as well, directly by improving the contraction of the IVS [168] and indirectly due to its 'wringing' action [331, 332] and, as such, poor LV systolic function may result in RV-F [170]. The RV contractility may be compromised [47, 69, 75, 88, 108] by a number of different conditions, including AMI involving the right ventricle [45, 108, 246] and PH from PE [12, 75, 101], sepsis [83, 147], and acute respiratory failure [59–62]. Thus, in life threatening situations and particularly where initial therapy is unsuccessful [249, 280–282, 284, 285] the use of inotropic drugs must be considered.

Dobutamine has been the agent of choice for some time [248, 330, 333] and is able to improve right (and left) ventricular contractility [14], right ventricular compliance [334], which will subsequently reduce RVEDP and RV wall stress, and it reduces the pulmonary resistance and thus RV-afterload [335, 336]. However; it is important to keep in mind the possible harmful effects with potentially unfavourable outcomes of dobutamine as mentioned in Chapter 2 [337–340].

Levosimendan has recently been shown to be effective in the treatment of RV-F and superior to dobutamine [70]. Kerbaul showed a significant reduction in PVR, in mean and diastolic PA-pressure, PCWP, as well as a significant improvement of SV, CI and RV/LV-SWI. The main beneficial mechanism identified was an unloading of the RV through pulmonary vasodilatation [70, 252]. Morelli [252] investigated the treatment of RV-F with levosimendan in patients suffering from ARDS and also showed that levosimendan induces a substantial dilatation of the pulmonary vasculature [341, 342], reducing the pulmonary pressure and hence the RV-afterload. Levosimendan also appears able to improve RV contractility [341, 343, 344] (aside from improving LV contractility) without increasing the myocardial oxygen demand and without impairing myocardial relaxation [345, 346]. Furthermore, there are two other beneficial effects that may have contributed to the favourable outcomes seen in the studies by Kerbaul [70] and Morelli [252]. Levosimendan improves the ventriculo-arterial coupling of RV and the pulmonary artery. The $E_a:E_{es}$ ratio of the RV to the pulmonary artery was normalised [70]. Levosimendan seems to be preferable also because it does not compromise (RV or LV) diastolic function, and in fact beneficial effects on relaxation have been found [347, 348].

If inotropic support is necessary, levosimendan would appear to be the preferable drug in RV-F, but it is important to reiterate that, due to its vasodilative effects, normovolaemia [349] and a sufficient blood pressure to guarantee a proper RCA perfusion are prerequisites before commencing levosimendan administration. If necessary, a combination with noradrenaline will be required [349–351].

### v)        Intra-aortic balloon pump

One of the main benefits of intra-aortic balloon counter pulsation is the **increase in diastolic perfusion pressure and coronary blood flow** [352–354] which plays a key role in the therapy of RV-F [158, 245, 250, 251, 286, 290–293, 355].

Jacobs [108] states that the IABP is known to be beneficial in the treatment of RV-F but, unfortunately, the IABP is underused and should be used more frequently in cases of RV-F [249].

### vi)       Hypercapnia and acidosis

Hypercapnia and acidosis always induce an increase in pulmonary vascular resistance [356, 357] and thus affect the RV-function through an increase in RV-afterload [358, 359]:

**Hypercapnia/acidosis → ↑ PVR and concomitant ↑ PA-pressure → ↑ RV-afterload**

Respiratory balancing with the use of **mild hyperventilation** is an effective measure to protect the RV from high afterload [358, 360]. A reduction of $pCO_2$ from 50 mm Hg (6.66 kPa) to 30 mm Hg (4.0 kPa) will reduce the PVR and thus the RV-afterload from 700 dyn × s × cm$^{-5}$ to 400 dyn × s × cm$^{-5}$ [358].

### vii)      Oxygen therapy

Regardless of the underlying pathology, oxygen administration reduces pulmonary pressure and increases CO in patients with pulmonary hypertension [361]. It is widely appreciated that alveolar and systemic arterial hypoxaemia contribute significantly to vasoconstriction of the pulmonary vasculature, particularly in diseases such as COPD, ARDS, interstitial pulmonary diseases, pulmonary embolism and extensive pneumonia [4, 362] which results in an increased RV-afterload. Under conditions of systemic arterial hypoxaemia **oxygen administration** will lead to vasodilatation of the pulmonary vessels, and as long as there is no manifest fixed pulmonary hypertension, will lower RV-afterload significantly [19, 363] and improve RV-function [19, 364]. Continuous application of oxygen is the only measure to have been shown to reduce mortality in this situation [19].

### viii)     AV sequential stimulation

In order to optimise RV-filling (and RVEDP), maintaining or even improving RV-function **AV-synchronous stimulation is essential** [164, 365–367]. Therefore, to maintain or to restore **sinus** rhythm (cardioversion, *Amiodarone*, temporary two-chamber pacemaker) is **pivotal** as a normal (physiological) atrial function is essential to optimise RV (LV) filling [367].

Furthermore, persistant bradycardia will have a negative effect on both LV and RV filling and, as such, atropine or temporary pacing should be used to prevent this [164].

### ix)    Mechanical ventilation

Mechanical positive pressure ventilation contributes to an increase in RV-afterload [35, 178, 181, 368] due to an increase in transpulmonary pressures [18, 30, 32, 33, 175, 176], potentially leading to a deterioration in RV-function [180, 312] (as described above). Mechanical positive pressure ventilation also increases the risk of DVI by raising the pleural and thus the pericardial pressure (PP) [94]. Therefore, intubation and ventilation with positive pressure support should be avoided in patients with RVD/RV-F, if possible [369]. If mechanical ventilation is essential then levels of PEEP should be controlled. PEEP up to a certain level (~ 10 cm $H_2O$), although causing an increase in transpulmonary pressure [36–39, 53, 177] and thus a rise in RV-afterload [178, 179], may improve the blood flow through the pulmonary vasculature [40, 184–186], resulting in a net reduction of the RV-afterload [184] at least as long as RV-F is not manifest [191]. Hence, if needed, mechanical ventilation with low tidal volumes and relatively low PEEP is appropriate in patients with pulmonary hypertension [16, 330], although Groeneveld [370] suggests that using high frequency oscillator ventilation avoids the problem of increasing afterload due to positive pressure.

### x)    Diuretics

Diuretics are indicated in volume overloaded patients who have a dilated RV with leftward shifted septum following initial stabilisation (maintenance of appropriate BP) of the circulation [330, 371]. Diuretics may induce metabolic alkalosis and thus aggravate hypoventilation and hypercapnia and, as such, should be used judiciously [372]. Moderate peripheral oedema should be tolerated [373, 374].

### xi)    Anticoagulation

In pulmonary hypertension, hypercoagulation in the pulmonary vasculature tree will always be present [375–377] and the development of micro-thrombi is highly likely [311]. Therefore, the use of heparin or LWMH in therapeutic dosage is indicated in all cases of pulmonary hypertension [376–379].

### xii)    Digoxin

Digoxin is potentially detrimental in two ways: inducing vasoconstriction in the pulmonary arterial system and altering venous return to the disadvantage of RV-SV [374], and therefore is not indicated in the treatment of RV-D/RV-F [380, 381].

## c)    Therapeutic conclusions

When the clinical picture suggests right heart dysfunction or failure it can be diagnosed most easily and practically by echocardiography [11, 14, 17, 18]. The most useful echocardiographic features are RV-dilatation / ↑ RVEDV, IVS leftward shift, TAPSE and a TR-jet of > 2.7 m/s [192, 201, 212, 213, 221–225]. Critically ill patients are at high risk of developing right heart failure [2, 12, 15–19, 47, 154] due to a temporary increase in pulmonary vascular resistance [15, 17, 18, 30, 31, 44, 52, 55, 57, 382–384, 385], often with sepsis being the main underlying reason for acute RV-F [68, 99, 319]. RV-F often then turns out to be the **crucial** (and sometimes final) **insult in acute critical illness** [2, 14, 17, 43, 152, 162, 386].

The pathophysiology is determined by PH [2, 18, 47, 266, 387] and the concomitant risk of RV myocardial ischaemia [18, 47, 48, 87, 152, 162]. Diastolic ventricular interaction [24, 25, 101, 107, 116, 117, 123–125], altered geometry of the RV with TR (auto) aggravating the haemodynamic dysfunction [79, 148] and with the series effect of LV and RV [106, 150] are other mechanisms involved. These may all combine to induce a vicious cycle leading to shock and MOF [18, 87, 152, 245, 290].

Therapeutic strategies have fundamentally changed in recent years, taking the underlying pathophysiology into account. Fluid administration is counterproductive in manifest RV-D and RV-F [14, 24, 51, 101, 116, 126, 146, 147] and may worsen the haemodynamic and clinical situation. Avoidance and treatment of RV-ischaemia [18, 108, 159, 245, 250, 251, 290] by sufficient coronary (RCA) perfusion pressure (which increases the net tissue perfusion) [158, 287–289, 291] and the critical reduction of PH [108, 246–249] are the key strategies in the therapeutic approach.

In fluid overload accompanied by significant RV-dilatation which is compromising the LV cavity size and filling [146, 147], it is a priority to reduce the volume load. In severely impaired RV systolic function, shock or life-threatening situations [14, 70, 246–248, 252, 294, 295, 332], inotropic support (levosimendan [70, 252]) along with vasopressors in case of hypotension – and thus low CCP [158, 286–289, 292–296] – should be provided, along with other supportive measures such as maintenance of sinus rhythm [267, 365–367] and relief of acidosis [358, 360].

## 4.6 Summary

## a) Summary of clinical features

**Definition:**
- **RV-D:** RVEDD/RVEDV ↑, RV-EF ↓, RV-SV **normal**
- **RV-F:** RVEDD/RVEDV ↑, RV-EF ↓, RV-SV ↓

**Appearance: RV-F (ESC-6):** → **Cold and Dry.**

Low output syndrome with ↑ **jugular venous pressure**, increased liver size, abdominal discomfort, renal failure, tachypnoea and hypotension, although BP may initially be preserved due to sympathetic-adrenergic reaction.

**Haemodynamic characteristics:** HR ↑/n/↓, sBP (initially n) ↓/↓↓, CI low (< 2.2 l/min/m²), ↑/↑↑ systolic and mean pulmonary pressure (PH), but PCWP low (< 12 mm Hg ), ↑/↑↑ RVEDP, no pulmonary congestion. Urine output: ↑/↓/n, hypoperfusion: ↑/↓/n, end organ hypoperfusion: ↑/↓/n.

**Diagnosis by echocardiogram:** RV-dilatation, leftward shift of IVS / paradoxical IVS, TAPSE ↓, TR-jet > 2.7 m/s.

**Aetiology:** Acutely exacerbated COPD, broncho-pulmonary diseases with hypoxic/hypercapnic pulmonary vasoconstriction, acutely decompensated chronic biventricular HF, acute/chronic

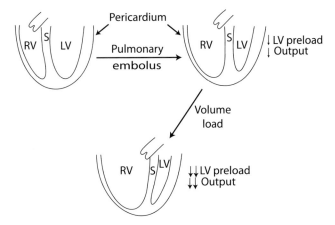

**Figure 4.2** Diagram adapted from Belenkie [116]. Acute RV loading causes RV dilatation, leftward septal deviation and DVI. This leads to a reduced LV-SV. Volume loading exacerbates this situation.

pulmonary embolism, acute RV-AMI, ARDS, mechanical ventilation, especially with "high" PEEP.

**Pathophysiology:** DVI, series-effect, autoaggravation and **ischaemia in the presence of pulmonary hypertension.**

## b)     Summary of treatment

- Treatment of **underlying disease:** Early thrombolytic therapy/PCI in case of acute coronary syndrome, thrombolytic therapy/catheter fractioning or embolectomy in pulmonary embolism, specific treatment of underlying broncho-pulmonary disease or sepsis.
- **Fluids:** Haemodynamic instability and life-threatening situations, in RV-D with normal PVR and in RV-AMI a well monitored fluid challenge is reasonable:
  CVP (before challenge) ≤ 9–10 mm Hg, *not increasing* by ≥ 2–5 mm Hg *during* fluid administration with positive effects: ↑ in RV-SV and LV-SV or sBP of ≥ 10%, improved peripheral circulation.
  In **RV-D** and in **RV-F no further fluid administration: Volume unloading** is appropriate at least in RV-F in order to stabilise and improve the patient's condition and increase SV/CO. In case of **fluid overload intravenous diuretics** are indicated after initial stabilisation.
- **Noradrenaline** to restore or maintain diastolic BP ≥ 60–65 mm Hg after preload is optimised or temporarily whilst adjusting preload.
- **Critical reduction of RV-afterload:** Bronchodilators in COPD/obstructive airways, inhaled pulmonary vasodilators such as NO/Iloprost; dosage NO is 10–40 ppm, Iloprost: recurrent inhalations of 10–20 μg over 10–15 min, sildenafil in stable patients, take care of possible systemic hypotension.
- Maintain or restore **AV sequential stimulation** (sinus rhythm), avoid/treat persistent bradycardia.
- $O_2$ **administration** in all cases.

- **Levosimendan** (take care of sufficient BP), in severely ↓↓ systolic RV function and/or ↓↓ systolic LV function.
- **Mild hyperventilation** if acidotic (pH < 7.2/7.1) or hypercapnic (> 6.7 kPa).
- **Avoid positive pressure ventilation** and **high PEEP** (> 10 cm $H_2O$) or use high frequency oscillator ventilation, if possible.
- Consider **IABP** at least in cases of inferior AMI or shock due to acute RV-F.
- Effective (therapeutic) **anticoagulation** is essential.

# Chapter 5

## Heart failure with normal left ventricular ejection fraction (HFNEF)

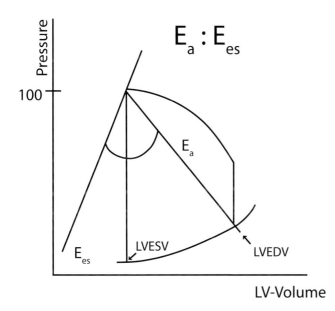

## 5.1    Definition

- Symptoms [1] and/or signs [2, 3] of heart failure, *and*
- Normal or mildly abnormal systolic LV-function (LV-EF > 50%), and
- Evidence of diastolic dysfunction.

There is considerable ongoing discussion about the term **diastolic** heart failure [4–6], with some authors demanding that this diagnosis be reserved for cases where an abnormality of the **intrinsic diastolic properties** [4, 7–11] of the heart is present. This is defined [12, 13] by a slowed relaxation and/or a decreased compliance (increased LV stiffness) characterising diastolic dysfunction [12, 13].

Diastolic dysfunction is not a unique finding in patients with diastolic heart failure but frequently occurs in patients with systolic LV dysfunction as well [14–18]. Many clinical conditions, myocardial as well as non-myocardial, are known to cause heart failure, including valvular heart disease, congenital heart disease, pericardial disease and right heart failure with normal systolic LV function [3, review by 7 and 19]. Abnormal diastolic function is the most common cause in these cases [7, 19].

The latest guideline from the ESC [1] uses the terms Heart Failure with Normal LV Ejection Fraction (HFNEF) and Heart Failure with Reduced LV Ejection Fraction (HFREF) and thus replaces the expressions diastolic heart failure and systolic heart failure.

## 5.2    Epidemiology and aetiology

Approximately 50% of all patients presenting with signs and symptoms of heart failure have a normal or only minimally impaired systolic LV function, thus suffering from HFNEF [20–25].

The prognosis of patients suffering from congestive heart failure with preserved systolic LV function was previously thought to be better than of those with reduced systolic LV-function [26] and indeed was supported by meta-analyses by Vasan [27] and by Thomas [28]. More recent estimates suggest that the prognosis in patients with HFNEF is as serious as those patients suffering from heart failure with impaired systolic function (HFREF) [29–33].

The main causes of an 'intrinsic' diastolic dysfunction and thus HFNEF are [2, 3, 5, 7, 12, 34]:

- (systolic) arterial hypertension [3, 13, 14, 35]
- coronary artery disease (CAD) [36]
- restrictive cardiomyopathy
- cardiac amyloidosis [3]
- genetically determined cardiomyopathy

Further predisposing factors have been identified [36–38]:

- increasing age and female gender [1, 35, 39]
- 60% of all patients suffer from diabetes mellitus [10, 11, 18, 35]
- 50% are obese [18]

- LV-hypertrophy [3, 40]
- elevated vascular stiffness [41–43]

These conditions have all been linked to ischaemia, fibrosis, and hypertrophy. All factors are able to induce abnormal relaxation and reduced LV-compliance [44] and diabetes may affect both the systolic as well as the diastolic function [45].

Systolic arterial hypertension is most commonly fundamental to the development of diastolic dysfunction and thus HFNEF [9, 12, 46, 47]. **Signs of diastolic dysfunction** in patients with **arterial hypertension mark the beginning of hypertensive cardiomyopathy** [48], and Vasan [27] found that nearly three quarters of all hypertensive patients presenting with heart failure had diastolic dysfunction as the underlying pathophysiology.

Non-hypertensive patients with signs and symptoms of heart failure generally have lower than normal blood pressures and a reduced cardiac output [5]. Abnormalities in diastolic properties limit the ventricle's ability to generate systolic pressure and stroke volume [40, 49]. Non-hypertensive patients with acute heart failure and preserved systolic function generally have marked concentric hypertrophy [40].

There is still an ongoing debate as to whether to classify HFNEF as a separate entity to HFREF in a two syndrome model or as a precursor of HFREF progressing to a significant impairment of systolic function. The latest ESC consensus guideline [1] addresses this debate.

Although beyond the scope of this chapter to recount all the details, the following facts should be stressed: There is now substantial evidence of structural [18] and functional [50] differences on the cardiomyocyte level between patients suffering from HFNEF and those with HFREF [18, 50]. Differing iso-form expressions of cytoskeletal proteins [51–53] and matrix metallo-proteinases [54–56] of the cardiomyocyte give profound reasons to classify HFNEF as a separate entity [49–55].

Baicu [57] was able to show with invasive studies that patients presenting with the typical signs and symptoms of congestive heart failure and initially diagnosed as suffering from diastolic heart failure had entirely normal systolic function. Hence, abnormalities of the diastolic function are responsible for the clinical picture in these patients.

Echocardiography [1, 7] remains the method of choice for assessment of heart failure, but increasingly we recognise that our diagnostic tools may not be sensitive enough to detect and measure the parameters which characterise HFNEF.

## 5.3    Pathophysiology

### a)    Abnormal relaxation and reduced LV compliance

Kitzman was the first to postulate an **abnormal, active relaxation and an elevated passive ventricular stiffness** present in patients with **diastolic heart failure** [13]. Zile [12] added further evidence to this patho-physiological view, thus summarising results gained by others [8–10, 19, 58, 59]:

Delayed (slowed) active relaxation and increased passive ventricular stiffness (reduced LV compliance as the inverse of chamber stiffness [19, 60]) **suggest abnormal diastolic function** [12].

Hence, **abnormal relaxation and reduced LV compliance** are the **hallmarks of diastolic dysfunction** [7, 12, 13, 59, 61]. Diastole in these patients may be prolonged, slowed or even incomplete [5, 34] and an altered relaxation will prolong the isovolumetric phase of the cardiac cycle and reduce the early diastolic filling (LVEDV ↓) [62, 63].

In most (or many [61]) patients suffering from HFNEF, both impaired relaxation and increased passive stiffness (decreased ventricular compliance) were found to be present [12, 64].

Whilst there is robust evidence that changes in the ventricular compliance undoubtedly account for the haemodynamic alterations and the patients' symptoms [5, 10, 13], until recently there was less evidence that abnormal relaxation alone could cause sufficiently significant symptoms [65, 66] along with pathological haemodynamics [6] (except in the case of tachycardia [67]). However, Leite-Moreira [68] provided clear **proof**, confirming indicative results by others [9, 42, 47, 69–72] that **prolonged ventricular relaxation** and **limited filling**, even if due to altered systolic loading conditions, **can translate into a substantial increase in LVEDP** and thus (acute) pulmonary oedema may occur [73, 74]. Furthermore, a delay in relaxation leads to a decrease in compliance, as Borlaug and Kass showed [75] and thus the abnormal left ventricular compliance (secondary to altered relaxation) may cause clinical and haemodynamic problems with the potential to induce pulmonary congestion or even pulmonary oedema [5, 10, 44, 76].

There is plenty of evidence that an elevated systolic ventricular load (afterload mismatch), such as that caused by an increase in systolic blood pressure or even an undetectable rise in intravascular and/or intraventricular volume, may induce acute heart failure with well preserved systolic function, particularly when there is elevated vascular stiffness and/or altered ventricular properties or deranged v-a coupling [9, 42, 43, 47, 68, 69, 71, 72]. In particular, Kawaguchi [47] showed that the diastolic ventricular function is affected by the arterial compliance. In response to reduced arterial compliance a concomitant reduction in cardiac compliance occurs [43, 47, 49]. Thus, a change in arterial conditions (due to a pressure rise or higher intravascular filling) may induce an inadequate rise in LVEDP [9, 47, 68] with the potential risk of pulmonary congestion as the first stage of pulmonary oedema [77] or even frank pulmonary oedema (see below).

Furthermore, LV relaxation is known to depend on end-systolic load and volume [78–82]. Hence, an increase in afterload affects both systole and (consecutive) diastole [42, 69, 83], and it is the **systolic conditions** rather than a primarily diastolic disorder that may lead to acute heart failure with **normal systolic function** [6, 9, 42, 43, 69].

Although patients with diastolic dysfunction may have a normal filling pressure (LVEDP) at rest [12, 61], the vast majority of them show **exercise intolerance** [61] as a typical marker of **altered diastolic properties** [6]:

- Kitzman [13] showed that there is a substantial rise in LVEDP during exercise. The pathophysiological mechanism taking effect is quite similar to that found in pulmonary oedema as described by Ghandi [9];
- The elevated LVEDP will reduce the pulmonary compliance and increase the respiratory work resulting in dyspnoea [12];
- An LV with reduced compliance has only a limited ability to utilise the Frank-Starling mechanism [13, 84]. This effect will be aggravated by the increase in heart rate during exercise, induc-

ing a shortening in the duration of diastole and thus the filling time of the stiff ventricle [13, 85, 86]. The overall result is an inadequate increase in SV for the situation [13, 84, 86].
- These pathophysiological findings and sequelae correlate well with the symptoms of exercise intolerance [12, 13, 84].

Thus, in patients with altered diastolic properties, a pathological elevation of LVEDP will be found in situations of (physiological) stress and will result in the symptoms of heart failure, as an elevated LVEDP is a trigger of cardiac dyspnoae [87, 88].

Tachycardia and particularly tachyarrhythmia may unmask subclinical diastolic dysfunction. A rapid heart rate shortens the diastolic filling period and the impaired diastolic relaxation results in an increase in LVEDP [13, 67, 85, 86]. Furthermore, in patients suffering from diastolic dysfunction the altered timing of systole and diastole (altered relaxation-frequency relation) results in an impairment of the a-v coupling as heart rate increases [89].

The main haemodynamic consequences of the abnormal diastolic properties are:

- ↑ in LVEDP [7, 12, 40, 48, 61, 86] (the diagnosis of HFNEF requires the presence of an elevated LVEDP [1, 2, 12, 61])
- Abnormal ventriculo-arterial coupling [47, 90]
- Inadequate or even no ↑ in SV during exercise (exercise intolerance) [12, 13]
- The left ventricular chamber size and volumes (LVEDV) are normal or even small [7, 11, 31, 86, 91]

## b)      Factors/mechanisms triggering development of acute heart failure

### i)      Ischaemia
Active ischaemia is known to impair diastolic relaxation [92]; silent ischaemia, caused by microvascular dysfunction [93, 94], is a particular problem in LVH with reduced coronary reserve [40]. There is an increasing oxygen demand in the case of arterial stiffening [95] which compromises diastolic function leading to acute HFNEF, and in the extreme case to flash pulmonary oedema [3].

### ii)      Abnormalities in afterload and ventriculo-arterial (v-a) coupling [9, 12, 21, 42, 47, 69, 96]
V-a coupling describes the interaction between ventricular and arterial properties and is an important determinant of cardiac performance [97–99] (see Chapter 1, 9d). In HFNEF, an abnormal interaction between the ventricle and arterial system is demonstrated, being the decisive pathophysiological mechanism in several clinical conditions [9, 13, 18, 47, 50].

- Vascular stiffness, expressed as $E_a$ (effective arterial elastance), rises due to age and hypertension [41, 42, 47], both are common in patients with HFNEF [3, 9, 40, 41]. The increase in $E_a$ is accompanied by a rise in ventricular systolic stiffness, expressed by $E_{es}$ [43, 47, 49, 100].

Normally, ventricular systolic properties match the vascular load in order to achieve optimal metabolic and mechanical conditions [101, 102] – thus, the consecutive increase in $E_{es}$ may be seen as a mechanism to achieve those goals [43].

- The cardiac properties at end-systole and the end-systolic volume are important determinants of early diastolic function [103, 104] and, as mentioned, LV relaxation depends on end-systolic load and volume [78–81]. Dys-synchrony of systolic contraction, i.e. due to altered systolic load, carries the risk of impairing diastolic function [70].

  Of note, an increase in $E_a$ increases myocardial oxygen consumption [95] with the potential risk of inducing ischaemia and further increasing the LVEDP;

- Abnormal end-systolic ventricular stiffness ($E_{es}$) is a common and characteristic finding in diastolic dysfunction [9, 12, 18, 44, 47, 50], particularly in patients with diseases affecting and altering primarily the (intrinsic) diastolic properties. Cardiac amyloidosis is a classical example of this [3]. The delay in LV-relaxation, characteristic of diastolic dysfunction [7, 12, 13, 59, 61], is accompanied by a prolongation of the mechanical systole in cases of altered diastolic properties [105,106]. Therefore, primarily systolic disorders will affect diastolic properties and vice versa [107, 108];

- In diastolic dysfunction – even if subclinical – a rise in afterload (i.e. increasing blood pressure, increase in circulating volume) causes a disproportional increase in $E_{es}$ and $E_a$ ($E_{es} > E_a$) which is called adverse or deranged v-a coupling [47, 90];

- Furthermore, high values of $E_{es}$ and $E_a$ augment systolic pressure sensitivity to cardiac loading conditions [9, 43, 96]. LV stiffness (reflected by an abnormal – high – $E_{es}$) in the presence of arterial stiffening is able to amplify the effects of changes in blood volume on systolic pressure and cardiac load – even a small increase in LV filling volume (LVEDV) leads to a disproportional rise in systolic blood pressure [43, 47]. This means an increase in systolic LV load and thus the concomitant increase in $E_{es}$ may induce a marked rise in LVEDP, provoking pulmonary oedema [43, 47, 96]. It is the increased left ventricular stiffness which makes the patient particularly vulnerable to developing pulmonary oedema [12].

It was Ghandi [9] who first postulated that a rise in systolic blood pressure (afterload rise) may increase LVEDP markedly, provoking rapid onset pulmonary oedema in patients with preserved systolic function. Hundley [42] provided strong evidence that reduced aortic distensibility ($E_a$ ↑) can cause heart failure presenting as flash pulmonary oedema. (Distensibility is a measure of compliance normalised to volume in order to compare different organs: Distensibility = C/V [60], C = compliance, V = volume). Najjer [69] concluded that even an acute rise in $E_a$, but with otherwise normal arterial elastance, might induce a substantial increase in LVEDP in the elderly with age-related higher $E_{es}$. Kawaguchi [47] impressively demonstrated that arterial stiffening in combination with ventricular stiffness may cause, due to deranged coupling, a prolongation of the LV relaxation and a restriction of LV-filling, the latter have both been shown to induce a substantial rise in LVEDP [68–72] leading to pulmonary oedema.

To summarise, the following factors/circumstances may cause, under the above described conditions, acute heart failure and even pulmonary oedema in patients with normal systolic LV function [3, 12, 31, 42–44, 47, 69, 92, 95, 109, 110]:

- increase in vascular resistance (i.e. rise in systolic blood pressure)
- volume load

- tachycardia
- ischaemia

Due to the importance of the vascular factors Bellot [109] and Little [110] stated that the development of acute heart failure, especially flash pulmonary oedema, in this large patient group should be seen as a **vascular** rather than a **cardiac** disorder.

This viewpoint is further supported by Burkhoff [6] and by Borlaug [75] who confirm that external (vascular) forces rather than intrinsic cardiac forces are able to induce acute heart failure.

## c)      Conclusion

The pathophysiological mechanisms causing acute heart failure with normal systolic function are obviously heterogenous [40, 64]. **Abnormal afterload** and **ventriculo-arterial mismatching** combined with **ischaemia** and **specific (intrinsic) diastolic disorders** of differing origins and their interaction can lead, via abnormal relaxation and impaired compliance, to a substantial rise in LVEDP and thus induce acute heart failure. This predominantly presents as acute pulmonary oedema, but with normal systolic function.

**Vascular abnormalities** ($\uparrow E_a$) resulting in **disturbed coupling between the ventricle and arterial system** and in alterations of the ventricular elastic properties may, when there are **acute changes** in blood pressure or volume conditions, cause an acute substantial rise in systolic LV load [9, 42, 43, 47, 69]. This leads to a prolongation of ventricular relaxation, impaired LV-filling and reduced LV compliance with the potential to induce a significant rise in LVEDP [68]. The induction of acute heart failure with normal systolic function (HFNEF) **in these circumstances** has obliged some authors to interpret the presence of pulmonary oedema **in the majority of patients admitted for HFNEF** as a **vascular disorder** rather than a cardiac one as it appears to be caused by an **acute afterload mismatch** occurring in the face of a pre-existing elevated $E_a$ (accompanied by an elevated $E_{es}$) and/or in the face of deranged v-a coupling [6, 75, 109, 110].

Whereas in the case of 'primarily' **intrinsic diastolic dysfunction** (cardiac amyloidosis or restrictive cardiomyopathy as classical examples) acute heart failure is a direct consequence of the primary increase in chamber stiffness (reduction of compliance) [12, 18, 44, 50], and it is this increase in left ventricular stiffness which makes the patient vulnerable to pulmonary oedema [12]. Thus, any additional insult such as ischaemia, exercise, new onset of atrial fibrillation or raised systolic blood pressure may lead, via the described mechanisms, to acute heart failure, often presenting as rapid onset pulmonary oedema.

## 5.4      Clinical features

## a)      Clinical appearance and general remarks

Typically, patients suffering from HFNEF are elderly women [111, 112] with arterial hypertension (with or without LV-hypertrophy), diabetes mellitus, and obesity [2, 3, 10].

In the hospital setting signs and symptoms of congestive heart failure are usually present, as many patients are hospitalised for decompensated HF or episodes of pulmonary oedema [1].

It is **essential** that all patients with acute heart failure undergo echocardiography in order to diagnose or exclude HFNEF or HFREF and, if the echo-result is suggestive of HFNEF, to aggressively seek underlying aetiologies and treat these appropriately [7].

As mentioned previously, the **obligatory criteria** in establishing the diagnosis of HFNEF as defined by the ESC [1] and others [2, 3] comprise:

1. Clinical signs of heart failure
2. Normal or near normal systolic function (EF > 50% [113, 114])
3. Evidence of abnormal relaxation and/or decreased compliance (indicated by either an **elevation of LVEDP in the presence of a normal or small LV chamber size** [2, 85, 115])

The combination of ↑ LVEDP and n/↓ LVEDV (LV chamber size) is essential to diagnose HFNEF [85, 115], although the finding of elevated cardiac pressures in a normal sized ventricle does not guarantee the clinical manifestation of diastolic (or systolic) dysfunction. This emphasises the integrated and multi-factorial nature of HF [49, 116], or to display congestive symptoms [117].

New onset of AF is frequent in HFNEF; the loss of the atrial contribution to LV-filling and the reduced time to fill may contribute to precipitate pulmonary oedema [118].

An elevated LVEDP in the presence of a normal or low LVEDV suggests an elevated chamber stiffness [7, 12] with the LV-distensibility reduced in such circumstances [1]. An abnormal increase in LVEDP with atrial contraction is suggestive of impaired compliance [119] and thus abnormal diastolic properties. Oh [7] describes that even a moderate decrease in LV compliance, equating to a moderate increase in chamber stiffness, will induce an abnormal increase in LVEDP and LAP.

Definitive objective evidence is required to diagnose abnormal diastolic properties [46, 109] and, if we follow recent publications [1, 3, 7, 27, 120–122], cardiac catheterisation is still seen as the gold standard in the diagnostic process:

↑ LVEDP (> 16 mm Hg [123]) **in the presence of** n/↓ LVEDV **and** normal LV-EF (> 50%)*

(* either obtained by echo or catheterisation [113, 114]).

Burkhoff [6] and Oh [7] state that an elevated LVEDP (> 16 mm Hg) in the presence of a normal sized LV provides proof of diastolic dysfunction if criteria 1 and 2 are fulfilled.

## b) Diastolic pressure-volume relation

The assessment of the **diastolic pressure-volume (P-V) relation** is the most accurate way to describe and evaluate cardiac diastolic properties [60] – but this invasive method is not feasible in daily practice as it involves fairly complex measurements of chamber stiffness at end-diastole with varying end-diastolic volumes [75]. The pressure-volume relation **during diastole** attempts to characterise the structural behaviour of the heart as a whole [60]. The relation is never linear, in general it is exponential [19].

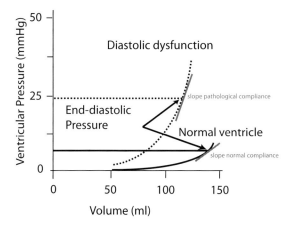

**Figure 5.1** Diastolic pressure-volume (P-V) relation – observe the different gradients of the slopes of the respective curves (modified from Westerhof et al. [125]).

**A steeper slope at the same position of an upward shifted pressure-volume relation gives proof of abnormal diastolic properties** [1, 6, 12, 44, 124].

In detail:

The ventricular **compliance** is reflected by the **end**-diastolic P-V relation. A **steeper slope** of the P-V curve at **end diastole** – steeper slope at the same position – **indicates elevated chamber stiffness and diminished LV-compliance respectively** [7, 125].

An ↑ in 'intrinsic' myocardial stiffness secondary to myocardial changes such as amyloidosis, fibrosis, etc., but also (transient) ischaemia result in a steeper slope of the P-V relation [126].

A slowed or incomplete ventricular **relaxation**, secondary to ischaemia (transient or sustained) or to 'intrinsic' abnormalities such as restrictive cardiomyopathy, LVH, etc, impairs the ability of the ventricle to accept volume loading [71, 120] with a **higher intraventricular pressure measured at any filling volume** [44] – upward shifted pressure-volume relation. Borlaug [75] also describes that a **delay in relaxation will decrease the ventricular compliance.**

**Figure 5.2** Abnormal relaxation (modified from Zile [127]).

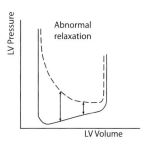

Parallel upward shifts of the P-V relation are not exclusively secondary to changes in diastolic properties [6]. Disorders of the pericardium [128], vascular abnormalities such as aortic stiffening [6, 75] or the cardiac constraining effects of raised intrathoracic pressure [129] may be revealed as well.

As discussed by Burkhoff [6] as well as by Borlaug and Kass [75] there are conflicting opinions as to how the P-V relation changes in HFNEF. While Zile [12] found a higher ventricu-

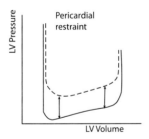

**Figure 5.3** Pericardial restraint (modified from Zile [127]).

lar stiffness and thus a change in LV compliance in HFNEF, the results by Kawaguchi [47], demonstrated in his study on arterial hypertension, are most accurately explained by a parallel upward shift of the pressure-volume relation. This is suggestive that external forces, including changes in aortic stiffness, are acting, which supports the 'vascular disease hypothesis' in these circumstances [109, 110].

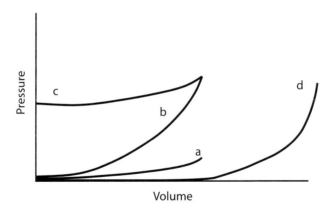

**Figure 5.4** Pressure-volume relation by Borlaug and Kass [75]: a: healthy humans; b: upward *and* leftward shift in diastolic dysfunction as described by Zile [12]; c: parallel changes as in pericardial disease described by Kawaguchi [47] in hypertensive patients with HFNEF; d: for comparison situation in dilated cardiomyopathy, typically demonstrating a rightward shift.

## c)    LV systolic function

EF is the most common parameter used to assess and express the systolic function of the left and right ventricles [130]. EF succeeds due to its easy application, is well understood, and its reliability to detect any abnormalities in contractility is at least reasonable [130]. The level of EF that defines a normal systolic function is somewhat arbitrary [131] but, nevertheless, in the current joint American and European echocardiography guidelines [132] as well as in the European Consensus statement on the diagnosis of HFNEF [1], a LV-EF > 50% determines a normal or only mildly impaired LV systolic function, as previously proposed by other authors [122, 133].

However, EF is far from being an ideal parameter to assess the contractility, and a preserved EF does not automatically imply normal systolic function [47, 134, 135]. Being depending on afterload, preload and on heart volume or mass [136–139], EF will fail to report excess afterload [140], in cases of augmented preload [141, 142] and when concentric LVH is present [143] (see Chapter 1, paragraph 6).

Often misinterpretation and a failure to detect an impaired systolic function can be avoided by assessing the longitudinal fibre shortening as well. The longitudinal shortening may be reduced but the EF appears to be normal or nearly normal secondary to an increase in the radial shortening compensating the longitudinal weakness [61]. Thus, the longitudinal shortening must be assessed separately in order not to miss a compromised systolic function [61]. A decrease in longitudinal shortening is an **early sign of LV (RV) systolic dysfunction** [144–146].

This can easily be done by assessing the systolic atrial-ventricular (AV) displacement of the mitral valve (systolic mitral valve annulus displacement) [135] or tricuspid valve (TAPSE), respectively. AV displacement reflects systolic LV (mitral valve annulus) and systolic RV (tricuspid valve annulus) function [147, 148]. Assessing the motion of the mitral valve annulus the subendocardial, **longitudinal** muscle fibres are examined [149]. Unfortunately, this element of contraction is not assessed by examining the ventricle in the conventional way [150] measuring the overall (global) performance in M- or 2D-mode, expressed by EF (or FS) [151]. The contribution to the global systolic function of the longitudinal fibres is normally greater than that of the circumferential fibres, which are usually assessed [152, 153].

Yip [150] showed that a significant number of patients with a normal EF, and therefore classified as suffering from HFNEF (in his study termed diastolic dysfunction), indeed have a reduced systolic function when assessing the longitudinal fibres by the mitral valve annulus displacement method.

The measurement is not only technically easy but it is shown to be markedly more sensitive than cardiac catheterisation and older echocardiographic parameters in detecting subtle systolic dysfunction [134, overview by 135, 149, 154–158].

Normal displacement amplitude of the mitral valve annulus is 12–14 mm [135, 155, 157–160]. A displacement of < 10 mm clearly indicates impaired systolic function [overview by 135] as well as an unfavourable prognosis [155, 161].

It should be mentioned that the velocity of the septal annulus site is usually lower than the lateral site, thus an average value of the measurements of both septal and lateral displacement is recommended for evaluation and decision making [1].

It was previously recommended that all patients should undergo echocardiography within 72 hours after onset of symptoms [2] in order evaluate the systolic function and in order to diagnose or exclude HFNEF because rapid improvement may be seen in a short time period. This appears redundant now as Ghandi [9] showed that no improvement of LV function can be expected in the days following hospitalisation, and thus there will be no change in systolic function on admission in comparison to a few days later. Expedient echocardiography is of course desirable for other reasons previously defined.

## d)   Echocardiographic parameters of diastolic dysfunction

The accuracy and sensitivity of echocardiography increasingly equals that of catheter techniques [1, 7] particularly if the recommendations of the American Society of Echocardiography and the European Society of Echocardiography [130] are followed. The use of the latest techniques, including tissue Doppler and the measurement/calculations of parameters such as E′, E/E′ ratio, pulmonary vein flow reversal, and left atrial volume index (LAVI), has increased the sensitivity greatly [1, 7, 37]. Echocardiography is non-invasive, portable, and its availability is still considerably higher than cardiac catheterisation; in fact, echocardiography is the most widely available and comprehensive diagnostic tool to identify such populations [7].

Several echocardiographic parameters are sensitive and reliable in reflecting diastolic properties and can be used in daily practice. These include isovolumetric relaxation time (IVRT) as defined by Wiggers [162], mitral valve deceleration time (mitral DT) determined by Doppler analysis of the mitral valve inflow patterns, E/A ratio of peak early (E) to peak atrial (A) Doppler mitral valve flow velocity, and pulmonary vein systolic and diastolic flow velocities [163–167]. However, all of these parameters have been the target of substantial criticism, and varying outcomes in regard to their predictive value have been found [168–172].

More recently, the combination of mitral inflow and pulmonary vein flow velocities has been suggested as having superior ability to assess diastolic function [37].

### i)        Difference between Ard time and Ad time

Diastolic dysfunction is suggested by abbreviated mitral inflow A-wave duration (Ad) (mitral inflow DT correlates well with PCWP when EF is reduced [173, 174]) and a longer duration of the flow reversal in the pulmonary veins (Ard) [7, 175, 176]. If the difference between Ard and Ad, is **more than 30 ms**, LV diastolic dysfunction can reliably be diagnosed [175–179].

### ii)       Tissue Doppler assessment

Furthermore, the Tissue Doppler (TD) assessment of the velocity of the mitral annular longitudinal myocardial fibre shortening and lengthening, called E′, has been a big step forward in the assessment of the diastolic properties of the LV. The lengthening velocity of the lateral and septal mitral annulus myocardial fibres in early diastole is considered to be a sensitive and reliable parameter reflecting diastolic properties [180, 181]. E′ is less influenced by loading conditions and other variables as compared to E [180, 182], and a reduction in E′ to < 8.0 cm/s [180, 183] clearly indicates a slowed relaxation [146]. Again, the combination of E and E′ is of special value. The E/E′ ratio estimates ventricular filling pressure (LVEDP) with good accuracy over a wide range of EFs [184–187]. Thus, with the ratio of the velocities of the E-wave of the mitral inflow patterns and the velocity of the E′ wave of the tissue Doppler assessment of the myofibres of the mitral valve annulus region, we are able to estimate the end-diastolic intraventricular left ventricular pressure (LVEDP) [184]:

- E/E′ > 15 → LVEDP > 15 mm Hg, and thus clearly elevated [184]
- E/E′ <  8 → LVEDP <  8 mm Hg (normal LVEDP) [184]

It must be remembered that, in cases of severe MR, the E/E′ ratio is not a reliable parameter with which to estimate LVEDP [188].

Ventricular compliance predominantly influences the LVEDP [189], but extracardiac factors may affect the LVEDP as well:

- Pulmonary pathologies, such as pneumonia or malignancy, can change the intrathoracic pressure and/or pressure in the pulmonary vascular system [190].
- Rising intra-abdominal pressure will increase the intraventricular pressure as well [191].

### iii)     LA volume index (LAVI)

LAVI and thus LA size [37] strongly reflects the severity and duration of diastolic dysfunction [192]. LAVI is relatively load-independent when assessing diastolic dysfunction [168] and LAVI > 40 ml/m$^2$ supports the diagnosis of diastolic heart failure [1].

### iv)     End diastolic LV volume (LVEDV)

An elevation of the LVEDP in the presence of normal or even small LV end-diastolic volumes is required to diagnose abnormal diastolic properties [2, 85, 115]. This requirement is based on the fact that LV relaxation is dependent on volume and systolic load as described above [79–82]. An LVEDVI > 97 ml/m$^2$ and an LVESVI < 49 ml/m$^2$ exclude any significant LV enlargement [1, 161].

### v)     Concentric LV hypertrophy

Concentric LV hypertrophy also has an impact on the diagnosis of HFNEF [11, 12, 18, 50, 133] and its presence may give direct evidence of abnormal diastolic properties [122]. An echocardiographically estimated LV wall mass index (LVMI) > 122 g/m$^2$ in women, > 149 g/m$^2$ men can give (see exclusion of HFNEF by the ESC criteria [1]) additional information, if needed.


Thus, the **echocardiographic indices**, recommended by the ESC [1], with which to assess the diastolic LV properties are:

- E/E' ratio (fundamental)
- Ard minus Ad
- LAVI
- E/A ratio and mitral DT
- LVMI

To assess the systolic function:

- **mitral annulus displacement**
- **conventional estimation of the LV-EF as described by Lang [132]**

Furthermore, of course, there is a need to **estimate the LV-size** in order to exclude LV enlargement and diagnose diastolic dysfunction [132].


Using **invasive left heart catheterisation**, a direct measurement of LVEDP > 16 mm Hg or a PCWP > 12 mm Hg, the latter measured by Swan-Ganz catheterisation, would suggest abnormal diastolic function. A LV relaxation time constant ($\tau$, Tau) of > 48 ms would support diastolic dysfunction but, as a prerequisite, a normal LVEDVI has to be present [186, 193–195].

## e)      Biomarkers

The measurement of **natriuretic peptides** may be helpful to support the diagnosis of HFNEF, but elevated levels are non-specific and do not provide sufficient evidence for diastolic dysfunction, and additional invasive (Tau) or non-invasive parameters are required [1, 196, 197].

NT-pro BNP was found to correlate well with early diastolic relaxation indices [196, 197], but NT-pro BNP and BNP do not exclusively reflect a distension of the LA and are found elevated in different conditions such as COPD [198], pulmonary embolism [199], and mechanical ventilation [200]. Furthermore, measurements of BNP/NT-pro BNP are not suitable to exclude preclinical diastolic dysfunction [201]. However, Tschope [197] confirmed results by Maisel [202] showing that NT-pro BNP/BNP have a **high negative predictive value** and, hence, normal values, in principle, rule out heart failure in general [197, 202].

Based on the above, the ESC consensus statement on the diagnosis of diastolic heart failure recommends the following approach [1]:

**HFNEF is excluded**, even if the patient's symptoms are suggestive of heart failure, when:
* There are no signs of fluid overload and a NT-pro BNP < 120 pg/ml (BNP < 100 pg/ml);
* Echocardiogram *excludes* valvular and pericardial disease and confirms LV-EF > 50% in the presence of:
    – LVEDVI < 76 ml/m$^2$ and
    – LAVI < 29 ml/m$^2$ and no atrial fibrillation (AF) and
    – LVMI < 96 g/m$^2$ (women), < 116 g/m$^2$ (men) and
    – E/E$'$ ratio < 8 and the peak systolic (S) shortening of LV basal (mitral) longitudinal myocardial fibre velocity > 6.5 cm/s.

**HFNEF is diagnosed** when:
* symptoms and signs of heart failure are present **and**
* LV-EF > 50% (mitral annulus displacement ≥ 12 mm) in the presence of a normal LV-size confirmed by LVEDVI < 97 ml/m$^2$ **and**
* evidence of diastolic dysfunction is confirmed by:
    – invasive measurement of LVEDP > 16 mm Hg / PCWP >12 mm Hg <u>and</u> τ >48 ms **or**
    – non-invasive (echocardiographic) measurements show:
        ♦ E/E$'$ > 15 or
        ♦ E/E$'$ > 8 but < 15, **and** NT-pro BNP > 220 pg/ml (BNP > 200 pg/ml) or
        ♦ – E/E$'$ > 8 but < 15, **and** atrial fibrillation or
            – E/E$'$ > 8 but < 15, **and** E/A < 0.5 and mitral DT > 280 ms or
            – E/E$'$ > 8 but < 15, **and** LAVI > 40 ml/m$^2$ or
            – E/E$'$ > 8 but < 15, **and** LVMI > 122 g/m$^2$ (women) / > 149 g/m$^2$ (men) or
            – E/E$'$ > 8 but < 15, **and** Ard minus Ad > 30 ms.

## 5.5      Therapeutic considerations

Unfortunately, there are no evidence-based strategies with which to manage patients suffering from HFNEF, due to the lack of trials in this area [3, 31, 64, 203]. Therefore, the therapy of HFNEF is empirical [203], based on the general principles of heart failure treatment.

In acute pulmonary oedema, the management described in Chapter 2 should be followed (GTN and, in confirmed fluid overload, a low dosage of diuretics [204–208]), as a reduction in afterload is the key aim [7, 9, 47, 42, 69].

Diuretics are widely recommended in fluid overloaded patients, diminishing breathlessness [3, 31, 203].

Due to abnormal diastolic function with impaired diastolic filling, drugs which reduce the heart rate and increase the duration of diastole, and hence the time for ventricular filling, are commonly used [3]. There is some evidence that rate lowering calcium channel blockers and β-blockers may be beneficial in the improvement of exercise tolerance and may reduce mortality as well [21]. Furthermore, β-blockers may protect against ischaemia (with its effects on ventricular compliance) and act to induce regression of hypertrophy [209, 210].

In patients with atrial fibrillation the restoration of sinus rhythm enables effective atrial contraction and aids filling of the LV having a beneficial effect [211].

**Good control of systemic blood pressure is** also **essential** [203] and inhibition of the renin-angiotensin system improves diastolic distensibility [212, 213]. Losartan induces a regression of LV hypertrophy and prevents further myocardial fibrosis [3, 214] as well lowering the LV afterload [215]. The LIFE-study [216], comparing losartan with atenolol, showed that the losartan group had less frequent cardiovascular complications. The CHARM study suggests a benefit in mortality with long-term administration of candesartan [217]. There are, however, inconsistent results in regard to a reduction in mortality when ACE-inhibitors are administered. A subgroup analysis of the V-HeFT trial [218] found some suggestion of a mortality lowering effect with the use of an ACE-inhibitor, but the CONSENSUS study [219] could not confirm this.

The Digoxin Investigation Group found no difference in mortality between HFNEF and HFREF patients, in both groups a similar reduction in hospitalisation was recognised [220].

## 5.6 Summary

About 50% of all patients suffering from (acute) heart failure have a normal or nearly normal systolic LV function. Whilst this was formerly termed diastolic heart failure, it is now more common to use the expression Heart Failure with Normal Ejection Fraction (HFNEF). HFNEF appears more common in elderly women with arterial hypertension along with those patients who are obese and/or diabetic. It is quite obvious that hypertension plays a key role and is probably the main cause for development of diastolic dysfunction in nearly three quarters of all hypertensive patients presenting with HFNEF.

Impaired relaxation and increased LV chamber stiffness are the characteristic elements of abnormal diastolic function; both are proven (relaxation with less evidence) to be able to increase LVEDP markedly, potentially provoking acute pulmonary oedema.

Vascular stiffening may cause a rise in end-systolic ventricular elastance and/or deranged v-a coupling can occur. This, together with an **acute afterload mismatch,** may lead to a **considerable rise in LVEDP** and the consecutive development of **flash pulmonary oedema.**

Post hoc study analysis supports the theory that external, namely **vascular forces/disorders** can act in raising the afterload and this interaction with the LV is an independent and **novel pathophysiological pathway in the development of acute heart failure with normal systolic function in a considerable number of patients.**

The diagnosis of HFNEF is confirmed if:

- signs and/or symptoms of heart failure are present,
- a normal or near normal systolic LV function is found and
- evidence of diastolic dysfunction is shown.

Abnormal diastolic function is suggested by an elevation of LVEDP (> 16 mm Hg) in the presence of a normal or even small LVEDVI (LV size).

An impaired LV compliance and thus compromised diastolic function is indicated by:

- a high LVEDP in the presence of a low LVEDVI,
- abnormal increase in LVEDP /LAP during diastole.

Although left heart catheterisation is still the gold standard for diagnosing diastolic dysfunction, echocardiography is more widely used and should be performed in all patients with symptoms of heart failure in order to try and identify the underlying aetiology. Mitral valve displacement analysis is technically easy and very sensitive in detecting even subtle systolic dysfunction.

Newer echocardiographic parameters are clearly more sensitive in detecting and reflecting diastolic abnormalities. The E/E' ratio is valuable in estimating LVEDP non invasively over a wide range of EF's and stands in the centre of the echocardiographic assessment and evaluation of diastolic ventricular properties.

Lacking sufficient specific studies, the therapy for HFNEF remains along the same lines as that for HFREF.

# References

## Chapter 1

1. Mohrman, DE and Heller, LJ   Cardiovascular Physiology, 4th edition. McGraw-Hill, 1997, pp 104–106
2. Burton, AC   Physical principles of circulatory phenomena. In: Handbook of Physiology Bd I/1 American Physiological Society, Washington, 1962
3. Weber, KT   J Appl Physiol 37 (1974): 742
4. Tan, LB   Cardiovasc Res 21 (1987): 615
5. Klabunde, RD   Cardiovascular Physiology Concepts. Lippincott Williams and Wilkins, 2005, http://www.cvphysiology.com/BloodPressure/BP012.htm
6. Kenny, L   Sports Med 1 (1984): 459
7. Scher, A   Textbook of Physiology: Circulation, Respiration, Body Fluids, Metabolism, and Endocrinology. PA. W. B. Saunders Co, Philadelphia, 1989, pp 972–990
8. Egan, B   Am Heart J 116 (1988): 594
9. Kumar, A   Crit Care 8 (2004): R 128
10. Michard, F   Chest 124 (2003): 1900
11. Cohn, JN and Franciosa, JA   NEJM 297 (1977): 27
12. Leier, CV   Current problems in Cardiology 21 (8) (1996): 527
13. Francis, GS   Pathophysiology of the heart failure clinical syndrome. In: Topol, E (ed) Textbook of Cardiovascular Medicine. Lippincott-Raven Publishers, Philadelphia, 1998, pp 2179
14. White, HD   Circulation 76 (1987): 44
15. Cotter, G   Europ J Heart Fail 5 (2003): 443
16. Fonarow, GC   Rev Cardiovasc Med 3 (suppl 4) (2002): S 41
17. Stevenson, LW   Am J Cardiol 66 (1990): 1342
18. Burton, AC   Am Heart J 54 (1957): 801
19. Woods, RH   J Anat Physiol 26 (1982): 302
20. Cohn, JN   Circulation 48 (1973): 5
21. Stevenson, LW   JACC 15 (1990): 174
22. Capomolla, S   Am Heart J 134 (1997): 1089
23. Rosario, LB   JACC 32 (1998): 1819
24. Otto, CM   NEJM 345 (2001): 740
25. Hamilton, MA   Am J Cardiol 65 (1990): 740
26. Moore, TD   Am J Physiol Heart Circ Physiol 281 (2001): H2385–H2391
27. Atherton, JJ   Lancet 349 (1997): 1720–1724
28. Dauterman, K   Ann Intern Med 122 (1995): 737
29. Stevenson, LW   Heart Fail 11 (1995): 87
30. Belenkie, I   J Appl Physiol 96 (2004): 917
31. Wells, RF   NEJM 270 (1964): 643
32. Kameyama, T   JACC 17 (1991): 199
33. Figueres, J   Am J Cardiol 44 (1979): 1349

34. ACC/AHA Task Force Guidelines for the Evaluation and Management of Heart Failure    JACC 26 (1995): 1376

35. Internat. AHA Guidelines Conference 2000    Circulation 102 (Suppl I) (2000): I-129 – I-135

36. Braunwald, E and Ross, J jr    Control of cardiac performance. In: Berne, RM, Sperclakis, N and Geiger, SR (eds) Handbook of Physiology: The Cardiovascular System Vol I. Williams and Wilkins, Baltimore, 1979, pp 533–580

37. Magder, S    The cardiovascular Management of the Critically Ill Patient. In: Pinsky MR (ed) Applied Cardiovascular Physiology. Springer-Verlag, Berlin, 1997, pp 28–35

38. Guyton, AC    Circulatory physiology: cardiac output and nits regulation. In: Guyton AC (ed), W. B. Saunders Co, 1973

39. Gould and Reddy (ed)    Vasodilatatory therapy for cardiac disorders. Futura, Mount Kisco New York, 1979, pp 1–6

40. Weber, KT    Am J Cardiol 47 (1981): 686

41. Katz, AM    Circulation 32 (1965): 871

42. Frank, O    Z Biol 32 (1895): 3703; (English translation: Am Heart J 58 (1959): 282)

43. Starling, EH    The Linacre Lecture on the Law of the Heart. Longmans Green &Co, New York, 1918

44. Asanoi, H    Circulation 65 (1989): 486

45. Belenkie, I    Ann Med 33 (2001): 236

46. Bleasdale, RA    Circulation 110 (2004): 2395

47. Holt, JP    Circ Res 8 (1960): 1171

48. Fewell, JE    Am J Physiol Heart Circ Physiol 240 (1981): H 821

49. Madger, S    Curr Opin Crit Care 12 (2006): 219

50. Klabunde, RD    Cardiovascular Physiology Concepts. Lippincott Williams and Wilkins, 2005, http://www.cvphysiology.com/CardiacFunction/CF006.htm

51. Glower, DD    Circulation 71 (1985): 994

52. Belenkie, I    Circulation 80 (1989): 178

53. Jardin, F    Am Rev Resp Dis 129 (1984): 135

54. Belenkie, I    Circulation 78 (1988): 761

55. Dupius, J    Am Heart J 120 (1990): 625-637

56. Holubarsch, C    Circulation 94 (1996): 683

57. Mirsky, I and Rankin    Circ Res 44 (1979): 601

58. Baker, AE    Am J Physiol Heart Circ Physiol 275 (1998): H 476

59. Tyberg, JV    Circulation 73 (1986): 428

60. Smiseth, OA    Am Heart J 108 (1983): 603-605

61. Traboulsi, M    Am Heart J 123 (1992): 1279

62. Boltwood, CM    JACC 8 (1986): 1289

63. Smiseth, OA    JACC 27 (1996): 155

64. McGeown, JG    Physiology. Churchill Livingstone, 2002, Chapter 3, p 71

65. Darovic, GO    Hemodynamic Monitoring: Invasive and non-invasive Application, 2nd edition. W. B. Saunders Company, Philadelphia, 1995

66. Alzeer, A    Can J Anaesth 45 (1998): 798

67. Kaltman, AJ    Circulation 34 (1966): 377

68. Falicor, RE    Circulation 42 (1970): 65

69. Bouchard, RJ    Circulation 45 (1971): 1072

70. Criley, JM and Ross, RS    Cardiovascular Physiology. Tarpon Springs, Florida, 1971

71. Hamilton, DR    Circulation 90 (1994): 2492

72. Smiseth, OA    JACC 23 (1994): 753

73. Stevenson, LW    Circulation 74 (1986): 1303

74. Grant, DA    Am J Physiol 266 (1994): H 2327

75. Grant, DA    Circulation 94 (1996): 555

76. Calvin, JE    Crit Care Med 9 (1981): 437

77. Cheatham, MC    Crit Care Med 26 (1998): 1801

78. Cullen, DJ    Crit Care Med 17 (1989): 118

79. Bristow, JD    Circulation 17 (1970): 219

80. Raper, R    Chest 89 (1986): 427

81. Eddy, AC    Am J Surg 155 (1988): 712

82. Michard, F    Chest 121 (2002): 2000

83. Kumar, A    Crit Care Med 32 (2004): 691

84. Böhm, M    Herzinsuffizienz. Thieme Verlag, 2000, pp 27

85. Janicke, JS    Fed Proc 39 (1980): 427

86. Tyberg, JV    Herz 15 (1990): 354

87. Grossman, W    Ann Intern Med 84 (1976): 316

88. Gilbert, JC    Circ Res 64 (1989): 827

89. Agostini, PG    Am J Cardiol 76 (1995): 793

90. Jardin, F    Chest 99 (1991): 162

91. Flessas, AP and Ryan, TJ    Circulation 65 (1982): 1203

92. Wood and Prewitt    Am J Cardiol 47 (1983): 963

93. Sibbald, WJ    Chest 84 (1983): 126

94. Alderman, EL    Circulation 54 (1976): 667

95. Humphrey, H    Chest 97 (1990): 11

96. Nohria, A    JAMA 287 (2002): 628

97. Fonarow, GC    Rev Cardiovasc Med 3 (suppl 4) (2002): S 18

98. Spotnitz    Circ Res 18 (1966): 49

99. Kampf, T    Der Internist 48 (2007): 899

100. Braunwald, E    Mechanisms of cardiac contraction and relaxation. In: Braunwald, E (ed) Heart Diseases. E. Saunders and Co, Philadelphia, 1988, pp 383–425

101. DeBacker, D and Minerva    Anesthesiol 69 (2003): 285

102. Sarnoff, SJ    Circ Res 8 (1960): 1077

103. Boehmer, RP    Crit Care Med 34 (2006): S 268

104. Madger, S    Shock Physiology. In: Pinsky, MR and Dhainhault, JF (eds) Physiological Foundations of Critical Care Medicine. Williams and Wilkins, Philadelphia, 1992, pp 140

105. Guyton, AC    Physiol Rev 35 (1955): 123

106. Magder, S    Venous return. In: Scharf, SM et al. (eds) Respiratory-circulatory interactions in health and disease. Marcel Dekker, New York, 2001, pp 93

107. Reddi, BAJ    J Appl Physiol 98 (2005): 356

108. Levy, MN    Circ Res 44 (1979): 739

109. Tyberg, JV and Pflügers    Arch Eur J Physiol 445 (2002): 10

110. Rowell, LB    Human Cardiovascular Control. New Oxford University Press, 1993

111. Shoukas, AA    Circ Res 33 (1973): 22

112. Scott-Douglas, NW    Can J Cardiol 18 (2002): 515

113. Scott-Douglas, NW    Am J Physiol 261 (1991): H 1693

114. Stephan, F    Am J Respir Crit Care Med 157 (1998): 50

115. Astiz, ME    Lancet 351 (1998): 1501
116. Landry, FH    NEJM 345 (2001): 588
117. Notarius, CF    Am Heart J 135 (1998): 339
118. Mirsky, MR and Payen, D    Crit Care 9 (2005): 566
119. Pinsky, MR    Chest 132 (2007): 2020
120. Mitchell, JP    Am Rev Respir Dis 145 (1992): 990
121. Levine, H    Med Conc Cardiovasc Dis 47 (1978): 95
122. Vieillard-Baron, A    Anesthesiology 94 (2001): 400
123. DeBacker, D    Int Care Med 33 (2007): 1111
124. Osman, D    Crit Care Med 35 (2007): 64
125. Michard, F    Am J Respir Crit Care Med 162 (2000): 134
126. Tavernier, B    Anesthesiology 89 (1998): 1313
127. Reuse, C    Chest 98 (1990): 1450
128. Calvin, JE    Surgery 90 (1981): 61
129. Bafaqueeh, F    Am J Respir Crit Care Med 169 (2004): A 344
130. Kroecker, CA    Am J Physiol Heart Circ Physiol 284 (2003): H 2247
131. Applegate, CP    Am J Physiol 262 (1992): H 1725
132. Finke, R    JACC 44 (2004): 340
133. Sourbrier, S    Int Care Med 33 (2007): 1117
134. Maizel, J    Int Care Med 33 (2007): 1133
135. Monnet, X    Crit Care Med 34 (2006): 1402
136. Wiedemann, HP    NEJM 354 (2006): 2564
137. Vincent, J-L and Weil, MH    Crit Care Med 34 (2006): 1333
138. Luecke, T    Crit Care 9 (2005): 607
139. Bendjelid, K    Int Care Med 29 (2003): 352
140. Connors, AF    NEJM 308 (1983): 263
141. Shippy, CR    Crit Care Med 12 (1984): 107
142. Marik, PE    Crit Care Med 29 (2001): 1635
143. Michard, F    Int Care Med 27 (2001): 1238
144. Eisenberg, PR    Crit Care Med 12 (1984): 549
145. Steingrub, JS    Chest 99 (1991): 1451
146. Mimoz, O    Crit Care Med 22 (1994): 573
147. Michard, F    Crit Care 4 (2000): 282
148. Reuter, DA    Br J Anaesth 94 (2005): 318
149. Grady, KL    Circulation 102 (2000): 2443
150. Stevenson, LW    JAMA 261 (1989): 884
151. Felker, M    Am Heart J 142 (2001): 393
152. Leier, CV    Prog Cardiovasc Dis 141 (1998): 207
153. Boulain, T    Chest 121 (2002): 1245
154. Lafaneclere, A    Crit Care 10 (2006): R 132
155. Taylor, RR    Am J Physiol 211 (1966): 674
156. Weber, KT    Am J Physiol 231 (1976): 337
157. Ilebekk, A    Scand J Clin Lab 39 (1979): 71
158. Thomas, M    Br Heart J 27 (1965): 17
159. Dark, PM    Int Care Med 26 (2000): 173
160. Lamia, B    Int Care Med 33 (2007): 1125

161. Preisman, S    Br J Anaesth 95 (2005): 746

162. Feissel, M    Chest 119 (2001): 867

163. Barbier, C    Int Care Med 30 (2004): 1740

164. DeBacker, D    Int Care Med 31 (2005): 517

165. Reuter, DA    Int Care Med 28 (2002): 392

166. Monnet, X    Int Care Med 31 (2005): 1195

167. Berkenstadt, H    Anesth Analg 92 (2001): 984

168. Tousignant, CP    Anesth Analg 90 (2000): 351

169. Hoeft, A    Anesthesiology 81 (1994): 76

170. Lichtwarck-Aschoff, K    J Crit Care 11 (1996): 180

171. Christakis, GT    Cardiovasc Surg 4 (1996): 29

172. Reuter, DA    Crit Care Med 31 (2003): 1399

173. Swanson, JD    Anesth Analg 83 (1996): 1149

174. Thys, DM    Anesthesiology 67 (1987): 630

175. Brock, H    Eur J Anaesthesiol 19 (2002): 288

176. Reuter, DA    J Cardiothorac Vasc Anesth 16 (2002): 191

177. Perel, A    Reanimation 14 (2005): 162

178. Slama, M    Am J Physiol Heart Circ Physiol 283 (2002): H 1729

179. Indra Singh and Pinsky, MR    Heart-Lung-Interaction. In: Papadakos, PJ and Lachmann, B (eds) Mechanical Ventilation: Clinical Applications and Pathophysiology. Saunders Elsevier, Philadelphia, 2008, pp 173–184

180. Coriat, P    Anesth Analg 78 (1994): 46

181. Reuter, DA    Br J Anaesth 95 (2005): 318

182. Fessler, H    J Appl Physiol 65 (1988): 1244

183. Brower, R    J Appl Physiol 58 (1985): 954

184. Pinsky, MR    Int Care Med 28 (2002): 386

185. Société de Réanimation    Reanimation 13 (2004): 253

186. Berkenstadt, H    Anesth Analg 92 (2002): 392

187. Bendjelid, K and Romand, J-A    Fluid responsiveness in mechanically ventilated patients: a review of indices used in intensive care. In: Pinsky, MR, Brochard, L and Mancebo, J (eds) Applied Physiology in Intensive Care Medicine. Springer, Berlin – Heidelberg, 2006, pp 95

188. Romand, JA    Chest 108 (1995): 1041

189. Fewell, JE    Cric Res 46 (1980): 125

190. Scharf, SM    J Appl Physiol 49 (1980): 124

191. Vieillard-Baron, A    Am J Respir Crit Care Med 168 (2003): 671

192. Jellinek, H    Crit Care Med 28 (2000): 672

193. Fessler, HE    Am Rev Respir Dis 146 (1992): 4

194. Braunwald, E    Circ Res 5 (1957): 670

195. Van den Berg, P    J Appl Physiol 92 (2002): 1223

196. Morgan, BC    Anesthesiology 27 (1966): 584

197. Vieillard-Baron, A    Anesthesiol 95 (2001): 1083

198. Vieillard-Baron, A    J Appl Physiol 87 (1999): 1644

199. Burton, AC    J Appl Physiol 12 (1958): 239

200. Culver, BH    J Appl Physiol 50 (1981): 630

201. Groeneveld, ABJ    J Appl Physiol 89 (2000): 89

202. Jardin, F    Anesthesiology 72 (1990): 966

203. Jardin, F    Circulation 83 (1983): 266
204. Robotham, JL    Crit Care Med 11 (1983): 783
205. Hanley, JA    Radiology 148 (1983): 839
206. Reuter, DA    Int Care Med 29 (2003): 476
207. Duperret, S    Int Care Med 33 (2007): 163
208. Perel, A    Anaesthesiology 89 (1998): 1309
209. Cariou, A    Crit Care Med 26 (1998): 2066
210. Boulnois, JL    J Clin Monit Comp 16 (2000): 127
211. Singer, M    Crit Care Med 17 (1989): 447
212. Valtier, B    Am J Respir Crit Care Med 158 (1998): 77
213. Bernardin, G    J Crit Care 13 (1998): 177
214. Goepfert, M    Int Care Med 33 (2007): 96
215. Laupland, KB    Can J Anesth 49 (2002): 393
216. Sinclair, S    BMJ 315 (1997): 909
217. Boulnois, JG    J Clin Monit 16 (2000): 127
218. Coyle, JP    Anesthesiology 59 (1983): A 53
219. Ornestein, E    J Clin Anesth 10 (1998): 137
220. Malbrain, ML    Crit Care Med 33 (2005): 315
221. Feissel, M    Crit Care Med 33 (2005): 2534
222. Berne, RM    Physiology, 4th edition. Mosby, St. Louis, 1998, pp 415–428
223. Chemla, D    Am J Physiol 274 (1998): H 500
224. Marx, G    Eur J Anaesthesiol 21 (2004): 132
225. DeBacker, D    Crit Care 10 (2006): 170
226. Pozzoli, M    Circulation 95 (1997): 1222
227. Takagi, S    Am Heart J 118 (1989): 954
228. Rocha, P    Crit Care Med 15 (1987): 131
229. Paelinck, BP    Eur J Echocardiogr 4 (2003): 196
230. Pittman, J    Crit Care Med 33 (2005): 2015
231. Linton, R    Br J Anaesth 86 (2001): 486
232. Kirov, MY    Crit Care 8 (2004): R 451
233. Sturm et al.    In: Lewis, FR and Pfeiffer, UJ (eds) Practical Applications of Fiberoptics in Critical Care
     Monitoring. Springer-Verlag, Berlin – Heidelberg – New York, 1990, pp 129–139
234. Eisenberg, P    Am Rev Respir Dis 136 (1987): 662
235. Mirsky, I    J Prog. Cardiovasc Dis 28 (1976): 277
236. Boussat, S    Int Care Med 28 (2002): 712
237. Simmons, RS    Am Rev Respir Dis 135 (1987): 924
238. Monnet, X    Int Care Med 33 (2007): 448
239. O'Rourke, MF    Arch Intern Med 144 (1984): 366
240. Magder, S    J Crit Care 14 (1999): 164
241. Pinsky, MR    Int Care Med 30 (2004): 1008
242. Madger, SA    J Crit Care 7 (1992): 76
243. Antonelli, M    Int Care Med 33 (2007): 575
244. Dellinger, RP    Crit Care Med 32 (2004): 858
245. Menon, V    JACC 36 (2000): 1071
246. Kern, JW    Crit Care Med 30 (2002): 1686
247. McConachie, I    Handbook of ICU Therapy, 2nd edition. Cambridge University Press, 2006, pp 29

248. Piene, H and Sund, T   Calculation of flow and pressure curves from the ventricular pressure-volume-time relationship and load impedance. In: T. Kenner et al (eds) Cardiovascular System Dynamics: Models and Measurements. New York Plenum, 1982, pp 47–56

249. Sakka, SG   Chest 122 (2002): 2080

250. Fernandez-Mondejar, E   J Crit Care 18 (2003): 253

251. Asfar, P   Intensive Care Med 33 (2007): 2045

252. Pfeiffer, KJ   Clin Intensive Care 5 (1994): 38

253. Bindels, A   Crit Care 4 (2000): 193

254. Katzenelson, R   Crit Care Med 32 (2004): 1550

255. Gödje, M   Europ J of Cardiothor Surgery 13 (1998): 533

256. Gödje, M   Crit Care Med 27 (1999): 2407

257. Sivak, ED   Crit Care Clin 2 (1986): 511

258. Bindels, AJ   Am J Cardiol 84 (1999): 115

259. Sakka, SG   Int Care Med 26 (2000): 180

260. Combes, A   Int Care Med 30 (2004): 1377

261. Bneditz, A   ESCIM congress 2003, abstract 60

262. Isakow, W   Am J Physiol Lung Cell Mol Physiol 291 (2006): L 1118

263. Takayama   Crit Care Med 19 (1991): 21

264. Halperin, BD   Chest 88 (1985): 649

265. Altschule, MD   Chest 89 (1986): 292

266. Raijmakers   Int Care Med 22 (1996): 591

267. Timmis, AD   BMJ 283 (1996): 591

268. Lichtwarck-Aschoff, J   Crit Care Med 18 (1992): 142

269. Bindels, A   Am J Cardiol 84 (1991): 1158

270. Oh, J   Am J Cardiol 66 (1990): 1492

271. Poelaert, JI   Chest 107 (1995): 774

272. Heidenreich, PA   JACC 26 (1995): 152

273. Weiss, RL   Chest 109 (1996): 73

274. Cigarroa, JE   NEJM 328 (1993): 35

275. Birmingham, GD   Am Heart J 123 (1992): 724

276. Come, PL   Chest 101 (1992): 151 S

277. Ritchie, JL   Circulation 95 (1997): 1686

278. Chaney, JC   Crit Care Med 30 (2002): 2338

279. Sakka, SG   J Crit Care 14 (1999): 78

280. Filipovic, M   Intensivemed 42 (2005): 13

281. Vieillard-Baron, A   Am J Respir Crit Care Med 166 (2002): 1310

282. Vieillard-Baron, A   Am J Respir Crit Care Med 168 (2003): 1270

283. Brown, JM   Crit Care Med 30 (2002): 1361

284. Price, S   Int Care Med 32 (2006): 48

285. Menon, V   Heart 88 (2002): 531

286. Porembka, DT   Transesophageal Echocardiography and Innovative Echocardiographic Technology. 1996

287. Vignon, P   Curr Opin in Crit Care 11 (2005): 227

288. Hüttmann, E   Acta Anaesthesiol Scand 48 (2004): 827

289. Vignon, P   Chest 106 (1994): 1829

290. Denault, AY   Can J Anaesth 49 (2002): 287

291. Schmidlin, D    Crit Care Med 29 (2001): 2143

292. Colreavy, FB    Crit Care Med 30 (2002): 989

293. Kaul, S    J Am Soc Echocardiography 7 (1994): 598

294. Fink, MP    Shock: An overview. In: Rippe et al. (eds) Intensive Care Medicine; Little and Brown, Boston, 1996, pp 1857–1877

295. LeDoux, D    Crit Care Med 28 (2000): 2729

296. Hochman, JS    NEJM 341 (1999): 625

297. Hollenberg, S    Ann Intern Med 131 (1999): 47

298. Bourgoin, A    Crit Care Med 33 (2005): 780

299. Varon, AJ et al.    Hemodynamic Monitoring. In: Civetta, JM et al. (eds): Critical Care, 2nd edition. J. B. Lippincott Co, Philadelphia, 1992, pp 255

300. Cheatham, ML    Crit Care Med 22 (1994): A 98

301. Eddy, VA    Chest 104 (suppl) (1993): 733

302. Nico, HJ    Circulation 92 (1995): 3183

303. Bourdarias, JP    Europ Heart J 16 (suppl I) (1995): 2

304. Meier-Hellmann, A    Intensivmed. 41 (2004): 583

305. Ruokonen, E    Crit Care Med 19 (1991): 1365

306. Bellomo, R    Am J Respir    Crit Care Med 159 (1999): 1186

307. Persson, PB    Curr Opin Nephrol Hypertens 11 (2002): 67

308. Bellomo, R    Crit Care 5 (2001): 294

309. Foster and Maes    Am J Physiol 150 (1947): 534

310. Navar, LG    Am J Physiol 274 (1998): F 433

311. Iglesias, J    Clinical Evaluation of Acute Renal Failure. In: Johnson, RJ (ed) Comprehensive clinical nephrology. Mosby, London, 2000: 15.4

312. Esson, MI    Ann Intern Med 137 (2002): 744

313. Chan, KHJ    Neurosurg 77 (1992): 55

314. Juul, N    Neurosurg Focus 11 (2001): 191

315. Artu, F    Neurol Res 20 (suppl 1) (1998): S 48

316. Bullock, RJ    Neurotrauma 17 (2000): 451

317. Cheatham, ML    Int J Crit Care Autumn (2000): 1–6

318. Torum, M    Congress of the Dep. Cardiology, University of Indonesia 29. Sep. 2005

319. Halperin, HR    Circulation 73 (1986): 539

320. Rivers, E    NEJM 345 (2001): 1368

321. Dellinger, RP    Crit Care Med 31 (2003): 946

322. Partick, DA    Am J Surg 184 (2002): 555

323. Carcillo, JA    Int Care Med 32 (2006): 958

324. Mythen, MG    Int Care Med 20 (1994): 99

325. Maillet, JM    Chest 123 (2003): 1361

326. Shoemaker, WC    Crit Care Med 27 (1999): 147

327. Shoemaker, WC    Crit Care Med 16 (1988): 1117

328. Beal, AL    JAMA 271 (1994): 226

329. Deitch, EA    Ann Surg. 216 (1992): 117

330. Goldberger, E    Essentials of Clinical Cardiology. J. B. Lippincott Comp, Philadelphia, 1990, pp 177

331. Miller, MJ    Anesth Analg 61 (1982): 527

332. Baele, AL    Anesth Analg 61 ( 1982): 513

333. Reinhart, K    Int Care Med 30 (2004): 1572

334. Pinsky, MR   Crit Care Med 33 (2005): 1119
335. Rady, MY   Am J Emerg Med 10 (1992): 538
336. Cain, SM   Am J Physiol 209 (1965): 604
337. Ronco, IJ   JAMA 270 (1993): 1724
338. Revelly, J-P   Crit Care Med 33 (2005): 2253
339. Henning, RJ   Circ Shock 9 (982): 307
340. Bloos, F and Reinhart, K   Venous oximetry. In: Pinsky, MR, Brochard, L and Mancebo, J (eds) Applied Physiology in Intensive Care Medicine. Springer-Verlag, Heidelberg, 2006, pp 37
341. De Backer, D   Lactic acidosis. In: Pinsky, MR, Brochard, L and Mancebo, J (eds) Applied Physiology in Intensive Care Medicine. Springer-Verlag, Heidelberg, 2006, pp 69
342. Ander, DS   Am J Cardiol 82 (1998): 888
343. Nakagawa, Y   Am J Respir Crit Care Med 157 (1998): 1838
344. Marik, PE   Crit Care Med 31 (2003): 81 B
345. Lima and J Bakker   Int Care Med 31 (2005): 1316
346. Groner, W   Nat Med 5 (1999): 1209
347. Liu, H   Med Phys 22 (1995): 1209
348. De Blasi, RA   Int Care Med 31 (2005): 1661
349. Andrews, P   Intensive Care Med 32 (2006): 207
350. Bakker, J   Chest 99 (1991): 956
351. De Backer, D   Am J Respir Crit Care Med 166 (2002): 98
352. Rady, MY   Am J Emerg Med 14 (1996): 218
353. Lush, CW   Micro Circulation 7 (2000): 83
354. Buwalda, M   Int Care Med 28 (2002): 1208
355. Tsoi, AG   Am J Physiol Heart Care Physiol 285 (2001): H 1545
356. Weber, KT   Fed Prog 39 (1980): 188
357. Weber, KT   Prog Cardiovasc Dis 24 (1982): 375
358. Grossman, W   J Clin Invest 56 (1975): 56
359. Gould, KL   Am J Cardiol 34 (1974): 627
360. Sandler, H   Circ Res 13 (1963): 91
361. Devereux, RB   JACC 17 (1991): 122
362. Braunwald, E   Heart Disease, 5th edition. W. B. Saunders Comp, Philadelphia, 1997, pp 421
363. McConachie, I   In: Handbook of ICU Therapy, 2nd edition. Cambridge University Press, 2006, pp 3–26
364. Westerhof, N, Stergiopulos, N and Noble, M   Snapshots of Hemodynamics. Chapter 17: Power and Efficiency. Springer Science and Business Media, Boston, 2005, pp 75
365. Westerhof, N, Stergiopulos, N and Noble, M   Snapshots of Hemodynamics. Chapter 23: Arterial Input Impedance. Springer Science and Business Media, Boston, 2005, pp 112
366. Westerhof, N, Stergiopulos, N and Noble, M   Snapshots of Hemodynamics. Chapter 26: Transfer of Pressure. Springer Science and Business Media, Boston, 2005, pp 131
367. Westerhof, N, Stergiopulos, N and Noble, M   Snapshots of Hemodynamics. Chapter 9: Law of La-Place. Springer Science and Business Media, Boston, 2005, pp 32
368. Rozich, JB   Circulation 86 (1992): 1718
369. Mirsky, I   Elastic properties of the myocardium.... In: Berne, RM (ed): Handbook of Physiology. Section 2, the Cardiovasc. System. Vol 1: The Heart. American Physiological Society, Bethesda, Md, 1979, pp 497–532
370. Reichek, N   Circulation 65 (1982): 99

371. Robinson, TF    Extracellular Structures in Heart Muscle. In: Harris, P and Poole-Wilson, PA (eds) Advances in Myocardiology. Plenum Publishing, New York, 1985, pp 243

372. Kolev, N    Transoesophgeal Echocardiography, a new monitoring technique. Springer-Verlag, 1995

373. Carabello, BA    Circulation 69 (1984): 1058

374. Rousseau, M    Circulation 62 (suppl III) (1980): III-91

375. Brutsaert, DL    Prog Cardiovasc Dis 16 (1973): 327

376. Nixon, JV    Circulation 65 (1982): 698

377. Borow, KM    Am J Cardiol 50 (1982): 1301

378. Weber, KT    Am J Cardiol 40 (1977): 740

379. Suga, H    Circ Res 35 (1974): 117

380. Sarnoff, SJ and Mitchell, JH    Am J Med 30 (1961): 747

381. Greim, C    Anaesthesist 44 (1995): 108

382. Grossman, W    Clinical measurements of vascular resistance and assessment of vasodilator drugs. In: Grossman, W and Baim, DS (eds): Cardiac Catheterization, Angiography and Intervention. Lea and Febiger, Philadelphia, 1991, p 143

383. Morita, SJ    Thorac Cardiovasc Surg 102 (1991): 774

384. Sunagawa, K    Am J Physiol 248 (1985): H 477

385. Lang, RM    Circulation 74 (1986): 1114

386. Kass, DA    Heart Fail Rev 7 (2002): 51

387. Nichols, WW    Circ Res 40 (1977): 451

388. O'Rourke, MF    J Hypertension 10 (1992): S 73

389. Sunagawa, K    Am J Physiol 245 (1983): H 773

390. Kelly, RP    Circulation 86 (1992): 513

391. Sunagawa, K    Circ Res 56 (1985): 586

392. O'Rourke, MF    Circ Res 20 (1967): 365

393. Taylor, MG    Circ Res 18 (1966): 585

394. Alexander, J    Am J Physiol 257 (1989): H 969

395. Shishido, T    Circulation 102 (2000): 1983

396. De Tombe, P    Am J Physiol Heart Circ Physiol 264 (1993): H 1817

397. Chemla, D    Am J Physiol Heart Circ Physiol 285 (2003): H 614

398. Baicu, C    Circulation 111 (2005): 2306

399. Maurer, M    J Card Fail 11 (2005): 177

400. Chen, C-H    JACC 32 (1998): 1221

401. Kelly, RP    Circulation 82 (suppl III) (1990): III-696

402. Ross, J jr    Prog Cardiovasc Dis 18 (1976): 255

403. Hausdorf, G    Intensivtherapie angeborener Herzfehler. Steinkopff, Darmstadt, 2000, pp 16

404. Cohn, JN    Am J Med 71 (1981): 135

405. Grossman, W    Cardiovas Res 13 (1979): 514

406. Carroll, JD    Circulation 67 (1983): 512

407. Zile, MR    NEJM 348 (2003): 735

408. Kaye, DM    JACC 23 (1994): 570

409. Steimle, AE    Circulation 96 (1997): 1165

410. Mehra, MR    Am Heart J 151 (2006): 571

411. Hundley, WG    JACC 38 (2001): 796

412. Leite-Moreira, AF    Cardiovasc Res 43 (1999): 344

413. Klabunde, RD    Cardiovascular Physiology Concepts, Lippincott Williams and Wilkins, 2005, chapter 4 pp 59 (especially p 81) http://www.cvphysiology.com/CardiacFunction/CF008.htm

414. Stevenson, LW   Am J Cardiol 60 (1987): 654
415. Braunwald, E   Heart Disease, 3rd edition. W. B. Saunders Comp, Philadelphia, 1988, p 413
416. Opie, LH   Mechanisms of cardiac contraction and relaxation. In: Braunwald, E (ed) Heart Disease, 7th edition. WB Saunders Company, Philadelphia, 2005, p 457
417. Bowditch, HP   Ber Sachs Ges Akkad 23 (1871): 652 and Arb Physiol Inst Lpz 6 (1871): 139
418. Schmidt, RF und Thews, G   In: Physiologie des Menschen, Springer-Verlag, 1977, p 378
419. De Tombe, PP   Am J Physiol 266 (1994): H 1202
420. Terkeurs, HE   Adv Exp Med Biol 226 (1988): 581
421. Karliner, J, K Peterson, and J Ross   Chapter 18. In: Braunwald, E (ed) Heart Disease, 3rd edition. W. B. Saunders Comp, Philadelphia, 1988, pp 188
422. Braunwald, E   Heart Diseases, 5th edition. 1997, p 430
423. Thys, DM   Advances in cardiovascular physiology. In: Kaplan, JA (ed) Cardiac Anaesthesia, 4th edition. Saunders Com, Philadelphia, 1998, chapter 7, pp 217
424. Quinones, MA   Circulation 53 (1976): 293
425. Mahler, F   Am J Cardiol 35 (1975): 623
426. Reeves, TG   Am Heart J 64 (1962): 525
427. Wallace, AG   Am J Physiol 205 (1963): 30
428. Furnival, CM   J Physiol (London) 211 (1970): 359
429. Yamada, H   J Am Soc Echocardiography 11 (1998): 442
430. Mehmel, HC   Circulation 63 (1981): 1216
431. Sagawa, K   Am J Cardiol 40 (1977): 748
432. Suga, H   Circ Res 32 (1971): 314
433. Grossman, W   Circulation 56 (1977): 845
434. Kass, DA   Circulation 76 (1987): 1422
435. Senzaki, H   Circulation 94 (1996): 2497
436. Sagawa, K   Circulation 63 (1981): 1223
437. Kass, DA   Eur Heart J 13 (suppl E) (1992): E 57
438. Talaoka, H   Circulation 87 (1993): 59
439. Braunwald, E   Heart Diseases, 5th edition. 1997, pp 432
440. Sodeman   Pathology Physiology. WB Saunders, 1974
441. Gomez, CM   Br J Anesth 81 (1998): 945
442. Braunwald, E   Heart Diseases, 5th edition. 1997, p 434
443. Mendoza, DD   Am Heart J 153 (2007): 366
444. Cotter, G   Curr Opin Cardiol 18 (2003): 215
445. Haas, GJ   Acute Heart Failure Management. In: Topol, EJ (ed) Textbook of Cardiovascular Medicine, 2nd edition. Lippincott, Williams and Wilkins, Philadelphia, 2002, pp 1856
446. Shah, MR   Europ J Heart Fail 4 (2002): 297
447. Morrow, DA   Circulation 102 (2000): 2031
448. Normand, SLT   JAMA 275 (1996): 1322
449. Lee, KL   Circulation 91 (1995): 1659
450. Jeger, RV   Chest 132 (2007): 1794
451. Saba, PS   J Hypertens 13 (1995): 971
452. Berne, RM and Levy, M   Cardiovascular Physiology. Mosby, 2001
453. Boron, W and Boulpaep, E   Medical Physiology: A cellular and Molecular approach. Elsevier/Saunders, Philadelphia, 2005
454. Borrow, KM   JACC 20 (1992): 787
455. Kreulen, TH   Circulation 51 (1975): 677

456. Gunther, S    Circulation 59 (1979): 679
457. Carabello, BA    Circulation 64 (1981): 1212
458. Zile, MR    JACC 3 (1984): 235
459. DeSimone, GJ    Hypertens 17 (1999): 1001
460. Mahadevan, G    Heart 94 (2008): 426
461. Devereux, RB    Am Heart J 146 (2003): 527
462. Devereux, RB    Hypertension 38 (2001): 417
463. Davies, M    Lancet 358 (2001): 439
464. McDonagh, TA    Lancet 350 (1997): 829
465. Pfeffer, MA    NEJM 327 (1992): 669
466. Cleland, SD    Eur Heart J 27 (2006): 2338
467. Niemienen, M    Eur Heart J 26 (2005): 384
468. Fonarow, GC    Rev Cardiovasc Med 4 (suppl 7) (2003): S 21
469. Gillebert, TC    Heart Fail Rev 5 (2000): 345
470. Grossman,W    Cardiac Catheterization and Angiography. Lea & Febiger, Philadelphia, 1980
471. Kawaguchi, M    Circulation 107 (2003): 714
472. Feldman, MD    Circulation 93 (1996): 474
473. Pak, PH    Circulation 98 (1998): 242
474. Silver, M    JACC 39 (2002): 798
475. Young, JB    Pharmacotherapy 16 (1996): 78 S
476. Abraham, T    JACC 46 (2005): 57
477. Capomolla, S    Europ J Heart Failure 3 (2001): 601
478. Burger, AJ    Am J Cardiol 88 (2001): 35
479. Ewy, GA    JACC 33 (1999): 572
480. Fonarow, GC    Rev Cardiovac Med 4 (suppl 7) (2003): S 21
481. Connors, AF    JAMA 276 (1996): 889
482. Sandham, JD    NEJM 348 (2003): 5
483. Fonarow, GC    Rev Cardiovasc Med 2 (suppl 2) (2001): S 7
484. Slawsky, MT    Circulation 102 (2000): 2222
485. Nieminen, MS    JACC 36 (2000): 1903
486. Jones, CS    Europ J Heart Fail 1 (1999): 425
487. Gomes, UC    Europ J Heart Fail 1 (1999): 301
488. Packer, M    NEJM 325 (1991): 1468
489. Moiseyev, VS    Russlan-Study. Europ. Heart J 23 (2002): 1422
490. Follath, F    Lido-Study. Lancet 360 (2002): 196
491. Zairis, MN    for the Investigators of the CASINO – Study ACC, 53rd Annual Scientific Session: Abstract 835-6. Presented March 9, 2004
492. Delle, KG    Acta Anaethesiol Scand 47 (2003): 1251
493. Revive-2-study    http://www.orion.fi/english/investors/stockreleases.shtml/a05?23290, 16. Nov. 2005
494. SURVIVE-study    http://www.orion.fi/english/investors/stockreleases.shtml/a05?23304,    16. Nov. 2005
495. Greenberg, B    Europ J Heart Fail 5 (2003): 13
496. Coletta, AP    Europ J Heart Fail 6 (2004): 673
497. Mebazaa, A    Am J Cardiol 95 (2005): 923
498. Ming, MJ    Shock 13 (2000): 459
499. Haikala, H    J Mol Cell Cardiol 27 (1997): 2155

500. Mulieri, LA   Circulation 85 (1992): 1743

501. Pieske, B   Circulation 92 (1995): 1169

502. Schwinger, RHG   Am Heart J 123 (1992): 116

503. Niehues   Herz-Kreislauf 9 (1977): 36

504. Fishberger, SB   Pacing Clin Electrophysiol 19 (1996): 42

505. Doval, HC   Lancet 344 (1996): 493

506. Marco, JP, Gersh, B and Opie, L   Chapter 8. In: Opie, L and Gersh, B (eds) Drugs for the Heart, 6th edition. Elsevier, 2005, pp 211

507. Santamore, WP   J Appl Physiol 41 (1976): 362

508. Janicki, JS   Am J Physiol 238 (1980): H 494

509. Bemis, CE   Circ Res 34 (1974): 498

510. Williams, L and Frenneaux, M   Nature Clin Pract Cardiovascular Med 3 (2006): 368

511. Glantz, SA   Circ Res. 42 (1978): 433

512. Badke, FR   Am J Physiol Heart Circ Physiol 242 (1982): H 611

513. Griggs, DM   Am J Physiol 198 (1960): 336

514. Laks, MM   Circ Res 20 (1967): 565

515. Belenkie, I   Am Heart J 123 (1992): 733

516. Ishihara, T   Am J Cardiol 46 (1980): 744

517. Kingma, I   Circulation 68 (1983): 1304

518. Gan, C   Am J Physiol Heart Circ Physiol 290 (2006): H 1528

519. Jardin, F   JACC 10 (1987): 1201

520. Olsen, CO   Circ Res 52 (1983): 85

521. Hoffman, EA   Am J Physiol Heart Circ Physiol 249 (1985): H 883

522. Lee, JM   Circ Res 49 (1981): 533

523. Ross, J jr   Circulation 59 (1979): 32

524. Shirato, K   Circulation 57 (1978): 1191

525. Rabkin, SW and Hsu, PH   Am J Physiol 229 (1975): 896

526. Zwissler, B   Anaesthesist 49 (2000): 788

527. Mebazza, A   Int Care Med 30 (2004): 185

528. Stoltzfus, DP   Anesthesiol Clin North Am 15 (1997): 797

529. Vonk-Noordergraaf, A   Chest 128 (2005): 628 S

530. Stojnic, BB   Br Heart J 68 (1992): 16–20

531. Calvin, JE   Circulation 84 (1991): 852

532. Dhainaut, JF   Int Care Med 14 (1988): 488

533. Schneider, AJ   Circ Shock 18 (1986): 53

534. Matthay, RA   Chest 101 (1992): 255 S

535. Jardin, F   Int Care Med 29 (2003): 361

536. Vieillard-Baron, A   Am J Respir Crit Care Med 166 (2001): 1481

537. Bunnell, IL   Am J Med 39 (1968): 861

538. Prewitt, RM and Ghignone   Crit Care Med 11 (1983): 346

539. Bleasdale, RA and Frenneraux, M   Heart 88 (2002): 323

540. Vieillard-Baron, A   Crit Care Med 29 (2001): 1551

541. Korr, KS   Am J Cardiol 49 (1982): 71

542. Mitchell, JR   Am J Physiol Heart Circ Physiol 289 (2005): H 549

543. Belenkie, I   Circulation 92 (1992): 546

544. Jardin, F   NEJM 304 (1981): 387

545. Menzel, T    Chest 118 (2000): 897

546. Mebazaa, A    The complex patient in the ICCU. Acute Cardiac Care Congress, 21st to 24th Oct 2006, Prague

547. Wiedemann, HP and Matthay, RA    Acute Right Heart Failure. In: Crit Care Clinics Vol 1 (No 3) 1985, pp 631

548. Mebazaa, A    Int Care Med 30 (2004): 185

549. Mercat, A    Crit Care Med 27 (1999): 540

550. Leschke, M    Der Internist 48 (2007): 948

551. Kimichi, A    JACC 4 (1984): 945

552. Stevenson, LW    Europ J Heart Fail 1 (1999): 251

553. Dec, W    JACC 46 (2005): 65

554. Freeman, G    J Clin Invest 86 (1990): 1278

555. Starling, MR    Am Heart J 125 (1993): 1659

556. Forrester, JS    Am J Cardiol 39 (1977): 137

557. Killip, T    Am J Cardiol 20 (1967): 457

558. Little, WC    Am J Physiol Heart Circ Physiol 261 (1991): H 70

559. Elzinga, G    Circ Res 68 (1991): 1495

560. Van den Horn, GJ    Circ Res 56 (1985): 252

561. Toorop, GP    Am J Physiol Heart Circ Physiol 254 (1988): H 279

562. Piene, H    Am J Physiol Heart Circ Physiol 238 (1980): H 932

563. Kass, DA    Ann Biomed Eng 20 (1992): 41

564. Sunagawa, K    Am J Physiol 56 (1983): 586

565. Piene, H and Sund, T    Am J Physiol 242 (1982): H 154

566. Yamakoshi, K    Jpn Circ J 49 (1985): 195

567. Milnor, WR    Circ Res 36 (1975): 565

568. Little, WC    Am J Physiol 253 (1987): H 83

569. Sugimachi, M    9th Conference on the Cardiovascular System Halifax, 1988, 227–230

570. Westerhof, N, Stergiopulos, N and Noble, M    Snapshots of Hemodynamics. Chapter 9: Law of La-Place. Springer Science and Business Media, Boston, 2005, pp 41

571. Asanoi, H    Circ. Res 65 (1989): 483

572. Borbley, A    Circulation, 111 (2005): 774

573. Van Heerebeek, L    Circulation 113 (2006): 1966

574. Grossman, W    NEJM 325 (1991): 1557

575. Zile, MR    NEJM 350 (2004): 1953

576. Ishihara, H    JACC 23 (1994): 406

577. Buckhoff, D    Am J Physiol 250 (1986): R 1021

578. Cohen-Solal, A    J Human Hypert 10 (1996): 111

579. Avolio, AP    Circulation 71 (1985): 202

580. Liu, CP    Circulation 88 (1993): 1893

581. Pak, PH    Circulation 94 (1996): 52

582. Ghandi, SK    NEJM 344 (2001): 17

583. Anjega, BG    Circulation 107 (2003): 659

584. Najjer, SS    JACC 44 (2004): 611

585. Ware, LB    NEJM 353 (2005): 2788

586. Straub, NC    Physiol Rev 54 (1974): 678

587. Brutsaerat, DL    Circulation 69 (1984): 190

588. Arieff, AI    Chest 115 (1999): 1371
589. Nussbacher, A    Am J Physiol 277 (1999): H 1863
590. Tan, LB    Postgrad Med J 67 (suppl 1) (1991): S 10
591. Williams, SG    Eur Heart J 22 (2001): 1496
592. Levine, TB    J Heart Lung Transpl 15 (1996): 297
593. Morley, D    Am J Cardiol 73 (1994): 379
594. Müller-Werdan, U    Cytokines and the Heart: Molecular mechanisms of septic cardiomyopathy. Landes, New York, 1996
595. Müller-Werdan, U    Intensivmed 43 (2006): 486
596. Müller-Werdan, U and Werdan, K    Septischer Kreislaufschock und septische Kardiomyopathie. In: Werdan, K, Schuster, H-P and Müller-Werdan, U (eds) Sepsis und MODS, 4th edition. Springer-Verlag, Heidelberg, 2005, pp 277–358
597. Herklotz, A    PhD-thesis at University Halle 2006
598. Poortmans, G    Transoesophageal echocardiographic evaluation of left ventricular function. In: Vincent, J-L (ed) Yearbook of Intensive Care and Emergency Medicine 1999. Springer, New York, 1999, p 468
599. Porembka, DT    Curr Opinin Crit Care 4 (1998): 195
600. DeBacker, D    Crit Care 10 (2006): 170
601. Bellot, JF    Causes and onset of pulmonary oedema. Acute Cardiac Care Congress 21st to 24th Oct 2006, Prague, reference 635
602. Little, WC    Hypertensive pulmonary oedema. Acute Cardiac Care Congress 21st to 24th Oct 2006, Prague, reference 636

# Chapter 2

1. Poole-Wilson, PA    Am J Cardiol 62 (1982): 31A
2. Nieminen, MS    Europ Heart J 26 (2005): 384
3. Forrester, JS    Am J Cardiol 39 (1977): 137
4. Killip, T    Am J Cardiol 20 (1967): 457
5. Cotter, G    Europ J of Heart Fail 5 (2003): 443
6. Adams, KF    Am Heart J 149 (2005): 209
7. Killip, T    Am J Cardiol 56 (1985): 2A
8. Strauer, BE    Der Internist 34 (1993): 912
9. Cleland, JGF    Europ Heart J 24 (2003): 442
10. Fox, KF    Europ Heart J 22 (2001): 228
11. Al-Khadra, AS    JACC 31 (1998): 749
12. Rudiger, A    Europ J Heart Fail 7 (2005): 662
13. Zannad, F    Europ J Heart Fail 8 (2006): 697
14. Klein, L    Ital Heart J 4 (2003): 71
15. Fonarow, GC    JACC (2004): 844
16. Paulus, WJ    Europ Heart J 28 (2007): 2539
17. Vasan, RS    Circulation 101 (2000): 2118
18. Angeja, BG    Circulation 107 (2003): 659
19. Burkhoff, D    Circulation 107 (2003): 656
20. Zile, MR    NEJM 350 (2004): 1953

21. Hogg, K   JACC 43 (2004): 317
22. Krumholz, HM   Arch Intern Med 157 (1997): 99
23. Fonarow, GC   Rev Cardiovasc Med 4 (suppl 7) (2003): S 21
24. Jong, P   Arch Intern Med 62 (2002): 1689
25. Owan, TE   NEJM 355 (2006): 251
26. Ross, J and Braunwald, E   Circulation 29 (1964): 739
27. Cohn, JN   Circulation 48 (1973): 5
28. Cohn, JN and Franciosa, JA   NEJM 297 (1977): 27
29. Francis, GS   Pathophysiology of the heart failure clinical syndroms. In: Topol, E (ed) Textbook of Cardiovascular Medicine. Lippincott-Raven Publishers, Philadelphia, 1998, pp 2179
30. Fonarow, GC   Rev Cardiovasc Med 3 (suppl 4) (2002): S 18
31. Straub, NC   Physiol Rev 54 (1974): 678
32. Leite-Moreira, AF   Cardiovasc Res 43 (1999): 344
33. Grossman, W   Cardiovas Res 13 (1979): 514
34. Carroll, JD   Circulation 67 (1983): 512
35. Kawaguschi, M   Circulation 107 (2003): 714
36. Ware, LB   NEJM 353 (2005): 2788
37. Ross, J jr   Prog Cardiovasc Dis 18 (1976): 255
38. Klabunde, RD   Cardiovascular Physiology Concepts, Lippincott Williams and Wilkins, 2005, http://www.cvphysiology.com/HeartFailure/HF 003.htm
39. Hausdorf, G   Intensivtherapie angeborener Herzfehler, Steinkopff, Darmstadt, 2000, pp 16
40. Cotter, G   Europ J of Heart Failure 4 (2002): 227
41. Mohr, R   Circulation 74 (1986): 780
42. Weil, J   Cardiovasc Res 37 (1998): 541
43. Ghandi, SK   NEJM 344 (2001): 17
44. Zampaglione, B   Hyperension 27 (1996): 144
45. Iriate, M   Am J Cardiol 71 (1993): 308
46. Brutsaerat, DL   Circulation 69 (1984): 190
47. Chen, C-H   JACC 32 (1998): 1221
48. Katz, AM   Circulation 73 (1986): III 184
49. Kass, DA   Heart Fail Rev 7 (2002): 51
50. Hundley, WG   JACC 38 (2001): 796
51. Avolio, AP   Circulation 71 (1985): 202
52. Little, WC   Europ Heart J 22 (2001): 1961
53. Pak, PH   Circulation 94 (1996): 52
54. Leite- Moreira, AF   Circulation 90 (1994): 2481
55. Kramer, K   Am Heart J 140 (2000): 451
56. Dodek, A   NEJM 286 (1972): 1347
57. Stevenson, LW   Am Heart J 135 (1998): 38
58. Nohria, A   JAMA 287 (2002): 628
59. Horwich, TB   Circulation 108 (2003): 833
60. Schrier, RW   NEJM 341 (1999): 577
61. Ferguson, DW   JACC 16 (1990): 1125
62. Gheorghiade, M   Circulation 112 (2005): 3958
63. Rosario, LB   JACC 32 (1998): 1819
64. Stevenson, LW   Am J Cardiol 66 (1990): 1348

65. Stevenson, LW    Circulation 90 (part 2) (1990): I- 611

66. Drazner, MH    J Heart Lung Transplant 18 (1999): 1126

67. Bindels AJGH    Am J Cardiol 84 (1999): 1158

68. Rotherbaum, DA    JACC 10 (1987): 264

69. Francis, GS and Archer, SL    J Intensive Care Med 4 (1989): 84

70. Yanci, CW    JACC 47 (2006): 76

71. Fonarow, GC    JAMA 293 (2005): 572

72. Gheorghiade, M    J Card Fail 11 (2005): 62

73. Gheroghiade, M    Am J Cardiol 96 (2005): 6A

74. Fonarow, GC    Circulation 90 (1994): I-488

75. Grady, KL    Circulation 102 (2000): 2443

76. Stevenson, LW    JAMA 261 (1989): 884

77. Hillege, HL    Circulation 102 (2000): 203

78. Nohira, A    J Card Fail 6 (2000): 64

79. Hochman, JS    NEJM 341 (1999): 625

80. Menon, V    JACC 36 (2000): 1071

81. Shamra, M and Terlink, JR    Curr Opinion in Cardiology 19 (2004): 254

82. Wang, CS    JAMA 294 (2005): 1944

83. Devereaux, RB    Hypertension 9 (1987): II-97

84. Bistrow, RB and Lowes, BD    Management of heart failure. In: Braunwald's Heart Disease. A Textbook of Cardiovascular Medicine, 7th edition. WB Saunders Company, 2005, pp 603

85. Nohria, A    JACC 41 (2003): 1797

86. Remes, J    Europ Heart J 12 (1991): 315

87. Cowie, MR    Europ Heart J 24 (2003): 1710

88. Maisel, AS    JACC 41 (2003): 2010

89. McCullough, PA    Am J Kidney Dis 41 (2003): 571

90. Cleland, JG    Curr Opin Cardiol 11 (1996): 252

91. Middelknauff, MR    Intern Med 37 (1998): 112

92. Stevens, TL    J Clin Invest 95 (1995): 1101

93. Brunner-La Rocha, H-P    J Hypertension 20 (2002): 1195

94. Levin, ER    NEJM 339 (1998): 321

95. Dao, Q    JACC 37 (2001): 379

96. Wang, TJ    NEJM 350 (2004): 655

97. Gardner, RS    Europ Heart J 24 (2003): 1735

98. HFSA    J Card Fail 9 (2003): S 79

99. Alpert, JS    JACC 36 (2000): 959

100. Jaffe, AS    Circulation 102 (2000): 1216

101. Newby, LK    JACC 41 (2003): 31 S

102. Heidenreich, PA    JACC 38 (2001): 478

103. Luscher, MS    Circulation 96 (1997): 2578

104. Sato, Y    Circulation 103 (2001): 369

105. Ishii, J    Am J Cardiol 89 (2002): 691

106. La Vecchia, L    J Heart Lung Transp 19 (2000): 644

107. Missov, E    Am Heart J 138 (1999): 95

108. Setsuta, K    Am J Cardiol 84 (1999): 608

109. You, JJ    Am Heart J 153 (2007): 462

110. Fincke, R   JACC 44 (2004): 340

111. Cotter, G   Chest 125 (2004): 1431

112. ACC/AHA Task Force Guidelines for the Evaluation and Management of Heart Failure   JACC 26 (1995): 1376

113. Blanke, H   Der Internist 34 (1993): 929

114. Frühwald, FM   Intensivmed. 35 (1998): 543

115. Felker, CM   Am Heart J 142 (2001): 393

116. Leier, CV   Prog. Cardiovasc Dis 41 (1998): 207

117. AHA/ACC guidelines   Circulation 100 (1999): 1016

118. DiDomenico, RJ   Ann Pharmacother 38 (2004): 649

119. Burton, AC   Am Heart J 54 (1957): 801

120. Abraham, WT   JACC 46 (2005): 57

121. Cheng, H   Europ Heart J Suppl 8 suppl E (2006): E 18 Review

122. Niemienen, M   Europ Heart J Suppl 8 suppl E (2006): E 6

123. Poole-Wilson, P and Opie, L   Chapter 6: Acute Inotrops: Sympathomimetics and Others. In: Opie, L and Gersh (eds) Drugs for the Heart, 6th edition. Elsevier, 2005, pp 150

124. Stevenson, LW   Europ Heart Fail 1 (1999): 251

125. Cardoso, J   Europ Cardiovasc Dis 1 (2006): 100

126. Dec, W   JACC 46 (2005): 65

127. Greenberg, B   Europ J Heart Fail 5 (2003): 13

128. Stevenson, LW   Am J Cardiol 60 (1987): 654

129. Woods, RH   J Anat Physiol 26 (1982): 302

130. Stevenson, LW   JACC 15 (1990): 174

131. Boehmer, RP   Crit Care Med 34 (2006): S 268

132. ACC/AHA guidelines   Circulation 104 (2004): 2996

133. Majid, PA   Lancet 2 (1971): 719

134. Mehra, M   Am Heart J 151 (2006): 571

135. Northbridge, D   Lancet 47 (1996): 667

136. Gheorghiade, M   Europ Heart J Supplements 7 (Supplement B) (2007): B 13

137. Peacock, WF   Rev Cardiovasc Med 3 (suppl 4) (2002): S 41

138. Pepine, CJ   J Clin Invest 64 (1979): 643

139. Franciosa, JA   Lancet 1 (1972): 650

140. Steimle, AE   Circulation 96 (1997): 1165

141. Weiland, DS   Am J Cardiol 58 (1986): 1046

142. Guhia, NH   NEJM 291 (1974): 587

143. Chatterjee, K   Circulation 48 (1973): 684

144. Atherton, JJ   Lancet 349 (1997): 1720

145. Packer, M   NEJM 235 (1991): 1486

146. Levine, HJ   JACC 28 (1996): 1083

147. Otto, CM   NEJM 345 (2001): 740

148. Deuterman, K   Ann Intern Med 122 (1995): 737

149. Wells, RF   NEJM 270 (1964): 643

150. Asanoi, H   Circ Res 65 (1989): 483

151. Internat. AHA Guidelines Conference 2000   Circulation 102 (Suppl I) (2000): I-129

152. Stevenson, LW   Circulation 108 (2003): 367

153. Capomolla, C   Am Heart J 134 (1997): 1089

154. Ruokonen, E   Crit Care Med 19 (1991): 1365

155. Bellomo, R    Am J Respir Crit Care Med 159 (1999): 1186

156. Lefer, AM    Fed Proc 37 (1978): 2734

157. Califf, RM    NEJM 330 (1994): 1724

158. Antman, EM    Acute myocardial infarction. In: Braunwald E, Fauci A, Kasper D et al. (eds) Harrison's Principles of Internal Medicine, 15th edition. McGraw-Hill, New York, 2001: 1395

159. Cotter, G    Lancet 351 (1998): 389

160. AHA/ Emergency Cardiac Care Committee    JAMA 268 (2002): 2199

161. Leier, CV    Am J Cardiol 48 (1981): 1115

162. Kelly, RP    Europ. Heart J 11 (1990): 138

163. Morrison, RA    Clin Pharmacol Th 33 (1983): 747

164. Menon, V    Am J Med 108 (2000): 374

165. Menon, V    Circulation 98 (suppl) (1998): I 630

166. Pulmonary Artery Catheter Consensus Conference    Crit Care Med 25 (1997): 910

167. Pulmonary Artery Catheter Education Project    http://www.pacep.org

168. Bernard, GR    JAMA 283 (2000): 2568

169. Williams, JF    Circulation 92 (1995): 2764

170. Partrick, DA    Am J Surg 184 (2002): 555

171. White, HD    Circulation 76 (1987): 44

172. Lim, H    Chest 124 (2003): 1885

173. Kohsaka, S    Arch Intern Med 165 (2005): 1643

174. Smith, HJ    Circulation 35 (1967): 1084

175. Cuffe, LS    JAMA 287 (2002): 1541

176. Adams, KF    Circulation 108 (Suppl IV) (2003): 695

177. Ewy, GA    JACC 33 (1999): 572

178. Carabello, BA    Circulation 105 (2002): 2701

179. Braunwald, E    Heart Disease, 5th edition. W. B. Saunders Comp, Philadelphia, 1997, pp 421

180. Mahadevan, G    Heart 94 (2008): 426

181. Devereux, RB    Am Heart J 146 (2003): 527

182. Devereux, RB    Hypertension 38 (2001): 417

183. Davies, M    Lancet 358 (2001): 439

184. McDonagh, TA    Lancet 350 (1997): 829

185. Pfeffer, MA    NEJM 327 (1992): 669

186. Cleland, SD    Eur Heart J 27 (2006): 2338

187. Fuhrmann, JT    Crit Care Med 36 (2008): 2257

188. Haque, WA    JACC 27 (1996): 353

189. Marcus, LS    Circulation 94 (1996): 3184

190. ACC/AHA-guidelines resuscitation    Circulation 102 (suppl II) (2000): I-172

191. Metha, RL    JAMA 288 (2002): 2547

192. Francis, GS    Ann Intern Med 103 (1985): 1

193. Young, JB    Pharmacotherapy 16 (1996): 78 S

194. Elkayam, U    Am J Cardiol 93 (2004): 237

195. Kloner, RA    JACC 42 (2003): 1855

196. Abrams, J    Am J Cardiol 77 (1996): 312

197. VMAC- Investigators    JAMA 287 (2002): 1531

198. Gottlieb, SS    Circulation 105 (2002): 1348

199. Kubo, SH    Am J Cardiol 60 (1987): 1322

200. Forrester, JS    NEJM 295 (1976): 1356

201. Loiacono, LA   Fluid resuscitation in the ICU. In: Higgins, Steingrub, Kacmarek and Stoller (eds) Cardiopulmonary Critical Care. BIOS Scientific Pub., 2002, pp 99

202. Philbein, EF   Am J Cardiol 80 (1997): 519

203. Cooper, HA   Circulation 100 (1999): 1311

204. Feldstein, C   Am J of Therapeutics 14 (2007): 135

205. Johnson, W   JACC 39 (2002): 1623

206. Jain, P   Am Heart J 145 (2003): 53

207. Krück, F   Drugs 41 (suppl) (1991): 60

208. Coppens, P   Clinical Reviews 102 (2002): 861

209. Chiariello, M   Circulation 54 (1976): 766

210. Zellner, C   Am J Physiol 276 (1999): H 1049

211. Protter, AA   Am J Hypertens 9 (1996): 432

212. Abraham, WT   J Card Fail 4 (1998): 37

213. Colucci, WS   NEJM 343 (2000): 246

214. Sharma, M   Current Opin in Cardiology 19 (2004): 254

215. Burger, AJ   J Cardiac Failure 5 (1999): 49

216. Burger, AJ   Am Heart J 144 (2002): 1102

217. Burger, AJ   Am J Cardiol 88 (2001): 35

218. Silver, M   JACC 39 (2002): 798

219. Busch, I and K. Werdan   in Madler, C (ed) Praktische Notfallmedizin, 2nd edition. Urban und Schwarzenberg, 1999, pp 441

220. Sakner-Bernstein, JD   JAMA 293 (2005): 1900

221. Dikshit, K   NEJM 288 (1973): 1087

222. Nelson, GIC   Lancet (1983): 730

223. Nieminen, M   Europ Heart J 7 (suppl 8) (2005): B 20

224. Wilson, JR   Am J Med 70 (1981): 234

225. Salvador, DR   Cochrane Database. Syst Rev 2005, issue 3, Art No: CD 003178. DOI: 10.1002/14651858.CD003718. pub3; and: http://www.cochrane.org/review/en/ab 003178.html

226. Neuberg, GW   Am Heart J 144 (2002): 31

227. Dormans, TP   JACC 28 (1996): 376

228. Sagar, S   Int J Clin Pharmacol Ther Toxicol 22 (1984): 473

229. Herlitz, J   Am J Cardiol 80 (1997): 40 J

230. Cody, R   JACC 22 (suppl a) (1993): 65 A

231. Cosin, J   Europ J Heart Fail 4 (2002): 507

232. Tsutamoto, T   JACC 44 (2004): 2252

233. Constanzo, MR   JACC 46 (2005): 2047

234. Bart, BA   JACC 46 (2005): 2043

235. Constanzo, M   UNLOAD TRAIL. Presented on the Congress of the American College of Cardiology 2006, March 13, Atlanta

236. Bart, BA   Heart Failure Society of America 2006 Scientific Meeting; September 11, 2006; Seattle, WA Abstract 375

237. Ali, SS   Heart Failure Society of America 2006 Scientific Meeting; September 11, 2006; Seattle, WA Abstract 374

238. Bart, BA   Heart Failure Society of America 2006 Scientific Meeting; September 11, 2006; Seattle, WA Comment on the study results in regard to Unload

239. Gheroghiade, M   Am J Cardiol 96 (suppl) (2005): 11 G

240. de Silva, R   Europ Heart J 27 (2006): 569

241. Mac Dowall, PA   Lancet 352 (1998): 13

242. Bongartz, LG   Europ Heart J 26 (2005): 11

243. Blake, P and Paganini, EP   Adv Ren Replace Ther 3 (1996): 163

244. Sharma, A   Cardiology 96 (2001): 144

245. Venkataram, R   Contrib Nephrol 132 (2001): 158

246. Mehta, RL   Therapeutic interventions in the cardiac intensive care unit: Dialysis and ultrafiltartion. In: Brown, DL (ed): Cardiac Intensive Care. Philadelphia, Saunders, 1998, pp 735–741

247. Connors, AF   JAMA 276 (1996): 889

248. Sandham, JD   NEJM 348 (2003): 5

249. Abraham, WT   J Card Fail 9 (suppl 1) (2003): S 81

250. Fonarow, GC   Rev Cardiovasc Med 2 (suppl 2) (2001): S 7

251. Sanborn, TA   JACC 36 (2000): 1123

252. Chen, EW   Circulation 108 (2003): 951

253. Anderson, RD   JACC 30 (1997): 708

254. Kern, MJ   JACC 21 (1993): 359

255. McGhie, AL   Chest 102 (suppl. 2) (1992): 626 S

256. Tuttle, RR   Circ Res 36 (1975): 175

257. Hollenberg, ST   Ann Intern Med 131 (1999): 47

258. Jaski, BE   J Clin Invest 75 (1985): 643

259. Fowler, MB   Circulation 74 (1986): 1290

260. Feldman, MD   Circulation 75 (1987): 331

261. Colucci, WS   J Clin Invest 81 (1988): 1103

262. Heino, A   Crit Care Med 28 (2000): 3484

263. Antman, EM   JACC 44 (2004): 671

264. McGhie, AL   Chest 102 (1992): 233

265. Leier, CV   Circulation 58 (1978): 466

266. Francis, GS   Am Heart J 103 (1982): 995

267. Hampton, JR   Lancet 349 (1997): 971

268. Stanchina, ML   Crit Care Med 32 (2004): 673

269. Dive, A   Int Care Med 26 (2000): 901

270. Thackray, S   Eur J Heart Fail 4 (2002): 515

271. Giraud, GD   J Pharmacol Exp Ther 230 (1984): 214

272. Van den Berghe, G   Crit Care Med 24 (1996): 1580

273. Capomolla, S   Europ J Heart Fail 3 (2001): 601

274. Martin, C   Chest 103 (1993): 1826

275. LeDoux, D   Crit Care Med 28 (2000): 2729

276. Müllner, M   Cochrane Database Syst Rev 2004, issue 3 Art No: CD 003709. DOI: 10.1002/14651858.CD003709. pub2; and: http://www.cochrane.org/review/en/ab003709.html

277. Martin, C   Crit Care Med 28 (2000): 2758

278. Levy, MM   Crit Care Med 33 (2005): 2194

279. Martin, C   Intensivmed 37 (2000): 507

280. Eckstein, J   Am Heart J 63 (1962): 119

281. DiGiantomasso, D   Int Care Med 28 (2002): 1804

282. Bersten, AD   New Horiz 3 (1995): 650

283. Bellomo, R   Am J Respir Crit Car Med 159 (1999): 1186

284. Vlahakes, G   Circulation 63 (1981): 87

285. DiGiantomasso, D   Chest 125 (2004): 2260

286. Meier-Hellmann, A   Int Care Med 22 (1996): 1354
287. Bohm, M   Europ Heart J 9 (1988): 844
288. Delle Karth, G   Acta Anaesthesiol Scand 47 (2003): 1251
289. Sakr, Y   Crit Care Med 34 (2006): 589
290. Colucci, WS   NEJM 314 (1986): 349
291. Alonsi, AA   Circulation 73 (1986): III-10
292. Shipley, JB   Am J Med Sci 311 (1996): 286
293. Lowes, BD   Int J Cardiol 81 (2001): 141
294. Bohm, M   JACC 30 (1997): 992
295. Packer, M   NEJM 325 (1991): 1468
296. Thackray, S   Eur J Heart Fail 2 (2000): 209
297. Felker, GM   JACC 41 (2003): 997
298. Terlink, JR   Heart Fail Monitor 4 (2002): 129
299. Haikala, H   J Cardiovasc Pharmacol 26 (suppl 1) (1995): S 10
300. Edes, I   Circ Res 77 (1995): 107
301. Pataricza, J   J Pharm Pharmacol 52 (2000): 213
302. Sonntag, S   JACC 43 (2004): 2177
303. Haikala, H   Idrug 3 (2000): 1199
304. Haikala, H   J Cardiovasc Pharmacol 25 (1995): 794
305. Hasenfuss, G   Circulation 98 (1998): 2141
306. Pagel, PS   Anesthesiology 81 (1994): 974
307. Jones, CS   Europ J Heart Fail 1 (1999): 425
308. Gomes, UC   Europ J Heart Fail 1 (1999): 301
309. Moiseyev, VS   Russlan-Study. Europ. Heart J 23 (2002): 1422
310. Follath, F   Lido-Study. Lancet 360 (2002): 196
311. Zairis, MN   Investigators of the CASINO – Study ACC, 53rd Annual Scientific Session: Abstract 835-6. Presented March 9, 2004
312. Packer, M   AHA Scientific Sessions 2005, Nov 13–16 Dallas, United States; now JAMA 297 (2007): 1883
313. Mebazaa, A   AHA Scientific Sessions 2005, Nov 13–16 Dallas, United States
314. Mebazaa, A   New therapies for acute heart failure. Presentation no 645 on the ESC congress Acute Cardiac Care, Prague 21st – 24th Oct 2007
315. Hermann, H-P   Intensivmed 41 (2004): 451
316. Delle Karth, G   Wien Klin Wochenschr 116 (2004): 6
317. Rabuel, C and Mebazaa, A   Int Care Med 32 (2006): 799
318. Slawsky, M   Circulation 102 (2000): 2222
319. Cleland, J   Curr Opin Cardiol 17 (2002): 257
320. Homes, J   Am J Cardiol 55 (1985): 146
321. Krahn, AD   Am J Med 98 (1995): 476
322. Doval, HC   Circulation 94 (1996): 3198
323. Kannel, WB   Am Heart J 115 (1988): 869
324. Benza, RL   J Cardiac Fail 10 (2004): 279
325. Pozzoli, M   JACC 32 (1998): 197
326. Unverferth, DV   Am J Cardiol 54 (1984): 147
327. Deedwania, PC   Circulation 98 (1998): 2574
328. Doval, HC   Lancet 344 (1994): 993
329. Singh, SN   NEJM 333 (1995): 77

330. Massie, BM    Circulation 92 (suppl I) (1995): I-143
331. Nul, DR    Circulation 92 (suppl I) (1995): I-666
332. Sharon, A    JACC 36 (2000): 832
333. Masip, J    Lancet 356 (2000): 2126
334. Peter, JV    Lancet 367 (2006): 1155
335. Naughton, MT    Circulation 91 (1995): 1725
336. Lenique, F    Am J Respir Crit Care Med 155 (1997): 500
337. Bersten, AD    NEJM 325 (1991): 1825
338. Lin, M    Chest 107 (1995): 1379
339. Kelly, CA    Europ Heart J 23 (2002): 1379
340. Pang, D    Chest 114 (1998): 1185
341. Bellone, A    Int Care Med 31 (2005): 807
342. Samama, MM    NEJM 341 (1999): 793
343. Kleber, FX    Am Heart J 145 (2003): 614
344. Barron, HV    Am Heart J 141 (2001): 933
345. Stone, GH    JACC 41 (2003): 1940
346. Boon, NA and Bloomfield, P    Heart 87 (2002): 395
347. Beling, M    Intensivmed 47 (2004): 12
348. Terlink, JR    Am Heart J 121 (1991): 1852
349. Rippe, JM    Acute Mitral Regurgitation. In: Rippe, JM et al. (eds) Intensive Care Medicine. Little,
     Brown and Company, Boston, 1985
350. Horstkotte, D    Akute Herzklappenfehler. In: Zerkowski, HR and Baumann, G (eds) HerzAkutMedi-
     zin, Steinkopff, Darmstadt, 1999
351. Grayburn, A    Am J Med Sci 320 (2000): 202
352. Hoit, BD    Curr Opin Cardiol 6 (1991): 207
353. Schon, HR    J Heart Valve Disease 3 (1994): 197
354. Kereiakes, JD and Ports, TA    Emergencies in valvular heart disease. In: Greenberg, BH and Murhpy,
     E (eds) Valvular Heart Disease, PSG Publishing Company, Littleton, 1986
355. Horstkotte, D, Loogen, F and Birks, W    Erworbene Herzklappenfehler. Urban and Schwarzenberg,
     1987
356. Rahimtoola, SH    Heart Dis Stroke 2 (1993): 217
357. Bonow, RO    Circulation 78 (1988): 1108
358. Greenberg, BH    Circulation 63 (1981): 263
359. Rapaport, E et al.    Aortic valve disease. In: Fuster, V (ed) Hurst's The Heart, McGraw-Hill, New York
     1994
360. Scognamiglio, R    NEJM 331 (1994): 689
361. Greenberg, B    Circulation 78 (1988): 92
362. Holtz, J    Intensivmed. 37 (2000): 644
363. Passik, CS    Mayo Clin Proc 62 (1987): 119
364. Khot, UN    NEJM 348 (2003): 1756
365. Awan, NA    Am Heart J 101 (1981): 386
366. Awan, NA    Br Heart J 39 (1977): 651
367. Germano, T    Valvular Heart Disease. In: Aghabahian, RV (ed) Emergency management in cardiovas-
     cular disease. Butterworth-Heinemann, Boston, 1994
368. Rahiamtoola, SH and Chandracatua, P    Valvular Heart Disease. In: Spittel JA (ed) Clinical Medicine
     Vol 6. Haper and Row Publishers, Philadelphia, 1983, pp 1–51

# Chapter 3

1. Fink, MP   Shock: An overview. In: Rippe et al. (eds) Intensive Care Medicine. Little and Brown, Boston, 1996, pp 1857-1877

2. Alpert, JS   Pathophysiology, diagnosis and management of cardiogenic shock. In: Blant, RC and Alexander, RW (eds) Hurst's The Heart: Arteries and Veins. Mc Graw-Hill, New York, 1994, p 907

3. Menon, V   Heart 88 (2002): 531

4. Francis, GS   Am Heart J 103 (1998): 995

5. Hochman, JS   NEJM 341 (1999): 625

6. Nohira, A   JAMA 287 (2002): 628

7. Tibby, SM   Arch Dis Child 28 (2003): 46

8. Menon, V   JACC 36 (2000): 1071

9. Menon, V   Am J Med 108 (2000): 374

10. Menon, V   Circulation 98 (suppl) (1998): I 630

11. Goldberg, RJ   NEJM 340 (1999): 1168

12. Hochman, JS   JACC 36 (2000): 1063

13. Steingrub, JS   Shock in Intensive Care Unit. In: Higgins, Steingrub, Kacmarek and Stoller (eds) Cardiopulmonary Critical Care. BIOS Scientific Pub., 2002, pp 81

14. Braunwald, E   Circulation 66 (1982): 1146

15. Heyndrickx, GR   Circ Res 72 (1993): 901

16. GUSTO-Investigators   NEJM 329 (1993): 673

17. ISIS- 3 Collaborative Group   Lancet 339 (1992): 753

18. The International Study Group   Lancet 336 (1990): 71

19. Babaev, A   JAMA 294 (2005): 448

20. Hands, ME   JACC 14 (1989): 40

21. GISSI Study Group   Lancet 328 (1986): 397

22. Goldberg, RJ   NEJM 325 (1991): 1117

23. Holmes, OR jr   JACC 26 (1995): 668

24. Goldstein, JA   JACC 19 (1990): 704

25. Gewirtz, H   Br Heart J 42 (1979): 719

26. Hochman, JS   Circulation 91 (1995): 873

27. Hochman, JS   Cardiogenic Shock. Annual Scientific Session, AHA – Dallas, TX, 1998

28. Scheidt, S   Am J Cardiol 26 (1970): 556

29. Killip, T   Am J Cardiol 20 (1967): 457

30. Hands, ME   JACC 14 (1989): 40

31. Leor, J   Am J Med 94 (1993): 265

32. Barron, HV   Am Heart J 141 (2001): 933

33. Hasdai, D   Eur Heart J 20 (1999): 128

34. Alpert, JS   Crit Care Clinics 9 (1993): 205

35. Blanke, H   Der Internist 34 (1993): 929

36. Hollenberg, S   Ann Intern Med 131 (1999): 47

37. McGhie, AI   Chest 102 (suppl 2) (1992): 626 S

38. Steingrub, JS   Cardiac Physiology. In: Higgins, Steingrub, Kacmarek and Stoller (eds) Cardiopulmonary Critical Care. BIOS Scientific Pub., 2002, pp 17

39. Califf, RM   NEJM 330 (1994): 1724

40. Greenberg, MA   JACC 13 (1989): 1071
41. Antman, EM   Acute myocardial infarction. In: Braunwald, E, Fauci, A, Kasper, D et al. (eds) Harrison's Principles of Internal Medicine, 15th edition. McGraw-Hill, New York, 2001, p 1395
42. Boehmer, JP   Crit Care Med 34 (Suppl) (2006): S 268
43. Cohn, JN   Circulation 48 (1973): 5
44. Francis, GS   Circulation 82 (1990): 1724
45. Cohn, JN and Franciosa, JA   NEJM 297 (1977): 27
46. Ross, J jr   Prog Cardiovasc Dis 18 (1976): 255
47. Cotter, G   Europ J Heart Failure 4 (2002): 227
48. Hochman, JS   Circulation 107 (2003): 2998
49. Geppert, A   Crit Care Med 30 (2002): 1987
50. Smith, HJ   Circulation 35 (1967): 1084
51. Cotter, G   Europ J Heart Fail 5 (2003): 443
52. Lim, H   Chest 124 (2003): 1885
53. Kohsaka, S   Arch Intern Med 165 (2005): 1643
54. Kohsaka, S   Circulation 104 (suppl II) (2001): II-483
55. Mitka, C   Shock 19 (2003): 305
56. Neumann, FJ   Circulation 92 (1995): 748
57. Prondzinsky, R   Der Internist 45 (2004): 284
58. Hochman, JS   Am Heart J 137 (1999): 313
59. Li, H   J Pathol 190 (2000): 244
60. Wildhirt, SM   Int J Cardiol 50 (1995): 253
61. Cotter, G   Europ Heart J 24 (2003): 1287
62. Müller-Werdan, U   J Mol Cell Cardiol 29 (1997): 2915
63. Lefer, AM   Fed Proc 37 (1978): 2734
64. Parrillo, JE   J Clin Invest 76 (1985): 1539
65. Nagy, S   Circ Shock 18 (1986): 227
66. Epstein, FH   NEJM 345 (2001): 588
67. Williams, SG   Heart 83 (2000): 621
68. Stevenson, LW   Circulation 108 (2003): 367
69. Nieminen, MS   Europ Heart J 26 (2005): 384
70. AHA/ACC guidelines   Circulation 100 (1999): 1016
71. Harizi, RC   Arch Intern Med 148 (1988): 99
72. Banka, VS   Am J Cardiol 34 (1974): 158
73. Miller, O   Br Heart J 68 (1958): 1614
74. Parker, JO   Arch Intern Med 129 (1972): 947
75. Figueras, J   Circulation 59 (1979): 955
76. Holubarsch, Ch   Circulation 94 (1996): 683
77. Ware, LB   NEJM 353 (2005): 2788
78. Braunwald, E   Circulation 66 (1982): 1146
79. Europ Study Group on diastolic heart failure   Europ Heart J 19 (1998): 990
80. Müller-Werdan, U   Europ Heart J 20 (suppl) (1999): 1721
81. Ruzumna, P   Curr Opin in Cardiol 11 (1996): 269
82. Jung, B   Heart 89 (2003): 459
83. Levine, RA   Circulation 112 (2005): 1817
84. Lamas, GA   Circulation 96 (1997): 827

85.  Pierard, L   NEJM 351 (2004): 1627

86.  Grossi, EA   Thoracic Cardiovasc Surg 16 (2001): 328

87.  Radford, MJ   Circulation 60 (suppl I) (1979): I-39

88.  Rahimtoola, SH   Heart Dis Stroke 2 (1993): 217

89.  Benotti, JR   Acute Aortic Insufficiency. In: Dalen, JE and JS Alpert (eds): Valvular Heart Disease, 2nd edition. Little, Brown and Co., Boston, 1987, pp 319

90.  Dervan, J   Acute Aortic Regurgitation: Pathophysiology and Management. In: Frankl, WS and Breast, AN (eds): Cardiovascular Clinics. Valvular Heart Disease: Comprehensive Evaluation and Management. FA Davis, Philadelphia, 1986, pp 281

91.  Oakley, CM   Heart 84 (2000): 449

92.  Bowles, NE   Curr Opin in Cardiology 13 (1998): 179

93.  Finkel, MS   Science 57 (1992): 387

94.  Balligand, J-L   J Clin Invest 91 (1993): 2314

95.  Rackley, CE   In: Chung, EK (ed) Cardiac Emergency Care, 4th edition. Lea and Febiger, Philadelphia, London, 1991, chapter 3, pp 36

96.  Oh, J   Am J Cardiol 66 (1990): 1492

97.  Poelaert, JI   Chest 107 (1995): 774

98.  Porembka, DT   In: Porembka DT (ed) Transesophageal Echocardiography and Innovative Echocardiography Technology. W. B. Saunders, Philadelphia, 1996

99.  Goldberger, E   Essentials of Clinical Cardiology. J. B. Lippincott Comp, Philadelphia, 1990, pp 177

100.  Monnet, X   Crit Care Med 34 (2006): 1402

101.  Ander, DS   Am J Cardiol 82 (1998): 888

102.  Wo, CCJ   Crit Care Med 21 (1993): 218

103.  Bland, RD   Crit Care Med 13 (1985): 85

104.  Rady, MY   Am J Emerg Med 10 (1992): 538

105.  Ryan, BP   Arch Emerg Med 8 (1991): 177

106.  Howell, MD   Int Care Med 33 (2007): 1892

107.  Wood, P   Diseases of the heart and Circulation, 2nd edition. Lippincott Co, 1956

108.  Forrester, JS   Am J Cardiol 39 (1977): 137

109.  Hasdai, D   Am Heart J 138 (1999): 21

110.  Lindholm, MG   Europ Heart J 24 (2003): 258

111.  Van de Werf, AD   Eur Heart J 24 (2003): 28

112.  Bertrand, ME   Europ Heart J 23 (2002): 1809

113.  McKee, S   Crit Care 11 (2007): 301

114.  Hall, AS   Lancet 343 (1994). 1632

115.  Wu, JP   Europ Heart J 14 (1993): 1273

116.  Kinch, JW   NEJM 330 (1994): 1211

117.  Stoltzfus, DP   Anesthesiol Clin North Am 15 (1997): 797

118.  Jacobs, AK   JACC 41 (2003): 1273

119.  Lee, FA   Cardiol Clin 10 (1992): 59

120.  Ross, J   Circulation 29 (1964): 739

121.  Piene, H and Sund, T   Am J Physiol 237 (1979): H 125

122.  Bellamy, RF   Am J Physiol 238 (1980): H 481

123.  Dell 'Italia, LJ   J Appl Physiol 78 (1995): 2320

124.  Feneley, MP   Circ Res 65 (1989): 135

125.  Sibbald, WJ   Crit Care Med 11 (1983): 339

126. Goldstein, JA  JACC 19 (1992): 704
127. Goldstein, JA  Circulation 82 (1990): 359
128. Molaug, M  Acta Physiol Scand 116 (1982): 245
129. Hines, R  Yale J of Biology and Medicine 64 (1991): 295
130. Banka, VS  Circulation 64 (1981): 992
131. Belenkie, I  Circulation 80 (1989): 178
132. Bleasdale, RA  Circulation 110 (2004): 2395
133. Kroecker, CA  Am J Physiol Heart Circ Physiol 284 (2003): H 2247
134. Mebazaa, A  The complex patient in the ICCU. Acute Cardiac Care Congress 21st to 24th Oct 2006, Prague
135. Goldstein, JA  JACC 2 (1983): 270
136. Dell 'Italia, LJ  Circulation 72 (1985): 1327
137. Love, JC  Am Heart J 108 (1984): 5
138. Francis, GS and Archer, SL  J Intensive Care Med 4 (1989): 84
139. Bindels, AJGH  Am J Cardiol 84 (1999): 1158
140. Rotherbaum, DA  JACC 10 (1987): 264
141. Raijmakers  Int Care Med 22 (1996): 591
142. Altschule, MD  Chest 89 (1986): 292
143. Takayama, Y  Crit Care Med 19 (1991): 21
144. Diamond, G  Circulation 45 (1972): 11
145. Calvin, JE  Crit Care Med 9 (1981): 437
146. Tousignant, CP  Anesth Analg 90 (2000): 351
147. Mirsky, I  J Prog.    Cardiovasc Dis 28 (1976): 277
148. Levine, H  Med Conc Cardiovasc Dis 47 (1978): 95
149. Kumar, A  Crit Care Med 32 (2004): 691
150. Michard, F  Chest 124 (2003): 1900
151. Katz, AM  Circulation 32 (1965): 871
152. Hust, MH  Intensivmed 42 (2005): 517
153. Tsuchihashi, K  JACC 38 (2001): 11
154. Dauterman, HL  Am J Cardiol 90 (2002): 838
155. Lee, L  Circulation 78 (1988): 1345
156. Verna, E  Europ Heart J 10 (1989): 958
157. Berger, PB  Circulation 99 (1999): 838
158. Hibbard, MD  JACC 19 (1992): 639
159. Hochman, JS  JAMA 285 (2001): 190
160. Urban, P  Europ Heart J 20 (1999): 1030
161. Hochman, JS  JAMA 295 (2006): 2511
162. Jeger, RV  Europ Heart J 27 (2006): 664
163. Webb, JG  Am Heart J 141 (2001): 964
164. Bengtson, JR  JACC 20 (1992): 1482
165. Antonicci, D  JACC 31 (1998): 294
166. Lemery, R  Am J Cardiol 70 (1992): 147
167. Calvo, EM  In: Braunwald (ed) Heart Diseases, 5th edition. Saunders and Co, Philadelphia, 1997, pp 1184
168. ACC/AHA guidelines  JACC 26 (1995): 1376
169. Woller, KC und Drexler, H  Der Internist 39 (1998): 459

170. ACC/AHA guidelines    Circulation 102 (suppl I) (2000): I-158

171. Tyivonni, D    Circulation 77 (1988): 392

172. Faber, TS    Drug Saf 11 (1994): 468

173. Trappe, H-J    Intensivmed 37 (2000): 724

174. Gibbons, R    NEJM 328 (1993): 685

175. Nico, HJ    Circulation 92 (1995): 3183

176. Bourdarias, JP    Europ Heart J 16 (suppl I) (1995): 2

177. Meier-Hellmann, A    Intensivmed. 41 (2004): 583

178. LeDoux, D    Crit Care Med 28 (2000): 2729

179. Bourgoin, A    Crit Care Med 33 (2005): 780

180. Halperin, G    JACC 44 (1999): E1

181. Vlahakes, G    Circulation 63 (1981): 87

182. Di Giantomasso, D    Int Care Med 28 (2002): 1804

183. Vincent, J-L and Weil, MH    Crit Care Med 34 (2006): 1333

184. Hunt, SA    JACC 38 (2001): 2101

185. Forrester, JS    NEJM 295 (1976): 1356

186. Boussat, S    Int Care Med 28 (2002): 712

187. Martin, C    Chest 126 (2004): 335

188. Cesare, JF    Circ Shock 39 (1993): 207

189. Berster, A    New Horizons 3 (1995): 650

190. Mathru, M    Chest 95 (1989): 1177

191. Ryan, TJ    Circulation 100 (1999): 1046

192. Giraud, GD    J Pharmacol Exp Ther 230 (1984): 214

193. Van der Berghe, G    Crit Care Med 24 (1996): 1580

194. DiGiantomasso, D    Chest 125 (2004): 2260

195. Sakr, Y    Crit Care Med 34 (2006): 589

196. ACC/AHA-guidelines resuscitation    Circulation 102 (suppl II) (2000): I-172

197. Silver, M    JACC 39 (2002): 798

198. Steingrub, JS    Cardiac Physiology. In: Higgins, Steingrub, Kacmarek and Stoller (eds) Cardiopulmonary Critical Care. BIOS Scientific Pub., 2002, pp 17

199. Willerson, JT    Am J Med 58 (1975): 183

200. Gacioch, GM    JACC 19 (1992): 647

201. Prewitt, RM    JACC 23 (1994): 794

202. Gurbel, PA    Circulation 89 (1994): 361

203. Anderson, RD    JACC 30 (1997): 708

204. Mueller, M    Circulation 45 (1972): 335

205. Bur, A    Rescuciation 53 (2002): 259

206. Papaioannou, TG    ASAIO J 51 (2005): 296

207. Torchina, DF    J Thor Cardiovasc Surg 113 (1997): 758

208. Ghali, WA    Ann Thorac Surg 67 (1999): 441

209. Antman, EM    Circulation 110 (2004): 82

210. Cowell, RP    Int J Cardiol 39 (1993): 219

211. Mehra, M    Am Heart J 151 (2006): 571

212. Shamra, M and Terlink JR    Curr Opinion in Cardiology 19 (2004): 254

213. Felker, CM    Am Heart J 142 (2001): 393

214. Leier, CV    Current problems in Cardiology 21 (8) (1996): 527

215. Böhm, M    Europ. Heart J 9 (1988): 844

216. Colucci, WS    NEJM 314 (1986): 290

217. Young, JB    Pharmacotherapy 16 (1996): 78 S

218. Abraham, T    JACC 46 (2005): 57

219. Capomolla, S    Europ J Heart Failure 3 (2001): 601

220. Lowes, BD    Int J Cardiol 81 (2001): 141

221. Jones, CS    Europ J Heart Fail 1 (1999): 425

222. Gomes, UC    Europ J Heart Fail 1 (1999): 301

223. Moiseyev, VS    .Russlan-Study. Europ. Heart J 23 (2002): 1422

224. Follath, F    Lido-Study. Lancet 360 (2002): 196

225. Coletta, AP    Europ J Heart Fail 6 (2004): 673

226. Cleland, JG    Europ J Heart Fail 6 (2004): 501

227. Edes, I    Circ Res 77 (1995): 107

228. Hasenfuss, G    Circulation 98 (1998): 2141

229. Haikala, H    Idrugs 3 (2000): 1199

230. Sonntag, S    JACC 43 (2004): 2177

231. Greenberg, B    Europ J Heart Fail 5 (2003): 13

232. Leather, HA    Crit Care Med 31 (2003): 2339

233. Yokoshiki, H    Europ J Pharmacol 333 (1997): 249

234. Kerbaul, F    Crit Care Med 34 (2006): 2814

235. SURVIVE-study    http://www.orion.fi/english/investors/stockreleases.shtml/a05?23304,    16. Nov. 2005

236. Mebazaa, A    New therapies for acute heart failure. Presentation no 645 on the ESC congress Acute Cardiac Care. Prague 21st – 24th Oct 2007

237. Cleland, J    Curr Opin Cardiol 17 (2002): 257

238. Slawsky, M    Circulation 102 (2000): 2222

239. Delle, KG    Acta Anaethesiol Scand 47 (2003): 1251

240. Hermann, H-P    Intensivmed 41 (2004): 451

241. Alhashemi, JA    Br J Anaesthesia 95 (2005): 648

242. Keh, D    Am J Respir Crit Care Med 167 (2003): 512

243. Annane, D    JAMA 288 (2002): 862

244. Dellinger, RP    Crit Care Med 32 (2004): 858

245. Confalonieri, M    Am J Respir Crit Care Med 271 (2005): 242

246. Kilger, E    Crit Care Med 31 (2003): 1068

247. Allolio, B    Clin Endocrinol 40 (6) (1994): 769

248. Woenckhaus, U    Intensivmed 42 (2005): 345

249. Forman, DE    JACC 43 (2004): 61

250. Akhter, MW    Am J Cardiol 94 (2004): 957

251. Fonarow, GC    JAMA 293 (2005): 572

252. Aronson, D    Am J Med 116 (2004): 466

253. Gheorghiade, M    Circulation 112 (2005): 3958

254. Gheorghiade, M    Am J Cardiol 96 (suppl) (2005): 11 G

255. Mehta, RL    JAMA 288 (2002): 2547

256. Sharma, A    Cardiology 96 (2001): 144

257. Metha, RL    Therapeutic interventions in the cardiac intensive care unit: Dialysis and ultrafiltration. In: Brown, DL (ed): Cardiac Intensive Care. Philadelphia, Saunders, 1998, pp 735–741

258. Shilliday, TR    Nephrol Dial Transplant 12 (1997): 2592

259. Mehta, RL    Crit Care 11 (2007): R 31

260. Neuberg, GW    Am Heart J 144 (2002): 31

261. Dormans, TP    JACC 28 (1996): 376

262. Sagar, S    Int J Clin Pharmacol Ther Toxicol 22 (1984): 473

263. Herlitz, J    Am J Cardiol 80 (1997): 40 J

264. Lassnigg, J    J Am Soc Nephrol 11 (2000): 97

265. Venkataram, R    Contrib Nephrol 132 (2001): 158

266. Lewis, J    Am J Kidney 36 (2000): 767

267. Blake, P and Paganini, EP    Adv Ren Replace Ther 3 (1996): 188

268. Al-Khafaji, A, Hampers, MJ and Crowin, HL    ACID-base disorders. In: Higgins, Steingrub, Kacmarek and Stoller (eds) Cardio-pulmonary Critical Care. BIOS Scientific Pub., 2002, pp 49

269. Mattar, JA    Am J Med 56 (1974): 162

270. Cooper, DJ    Ann Intern Med 112 (1990): 492

271. Bersin, RM    Circulation 77 (1988): 227

272. Shapiro, JI    Am J Physiol 258 (1990): H 1835

273. Forsythe, SM    Chest 117 (2000): 260

274. Nahas, GG    Drugs 55 (1998): 191

275. AHA-Statement    JAMA 268 (1992): 781

276. Kette, F    Crit Care Med 21 (1993): 901

277. Robertson, C    Resuscitation 37 (1998): 81

278. Hodgetts, T and Castle, N    In: Rescuscitation Rules. BMJ 1999, pp 52–54

279. Weisfeldt, ML    JAMA 266 (1991): 2129

280. Bruhn, HD    Niedrig dosiertes Heparin. Schattauer, 1996, pp 54–61

281. Stratton, JR    Circulation 75 (1987): 1004

282. Cregler, LL    Am Heart J 123 (1992): 1110

283. De Raffaele, C    Europ Heart J 28 (2007): 880

284. Kleber, XF    Am Heart J 145 (2003): 614

285. Levy, MM    Crit Care Med 33 (2005): 2194

286. Müllner, M    Cochrane Database Syst Rev 2004, issue 3, Art No: CD 003709. DOI: 10.1002/14651858.CD003709. pub2; and: http://www.cochrane.org/review/en/ab003709.html

287. Martin, C    Crit Care Med 28 (2000): 2758

288. Cheng, H    Europ Heart J Suppl 8 suppl E (2006): E 18

289. Reuter, DA    Crit Care Med 31 (2003): 1399

290. Coriat, P    Anesth Analg 78 (1994): 46

291. Tavernier, B    Anesthesiology 89 (1998): 1313

292. Reuter, DA    Br J Anaesth 95 (2005): 318

293. Preisman, S    Br J Anaesth 95 (2005): 746

294. Constanzo, M    presented on the Congress of the American College of Cardiology 2006, March 13, Atlanta

# Chapter 4

1. Raabe, DS    Chest 73 (1978): 96

2. Wiedemann, HP and Matthay, RA    Acute Right Heart Failure. In: Crit Care Clinics, Vol 1 (No 3). 1985, pp 631

3. Vincent, JL    Crit Care Med 22 (1994): 2024
4. Fishman, AP    Am Rev Respir Dis 114 (1978): 775
5. Weitzenbaum    Heart 89 (2003): 225
6. Rubin, LJ    Chest 126 (2004): 7 S
7. Chemla, D    Eur Respir J 20 (2002): 1314
8. Barst, RJ    JACC 43 (2004): 40 S
9. Galie`, N    Europ Heart J 25 (2004): 2243
10. Faber, HW    NEJM 351 (2004): 1655
11. Vieillard-Baron, A    Int Care Med 27 (2001): 1481
12. Vieillard-Baron, A    Am J Respir Crit Care Med 166 (2002): 1310
13. Health Central    http://www.healthcentral.com/mhc/top/000154.cfm, accessed June 2002
14. Mebazaa, A    Int Care Med 30 (2004): 185
15. Kannel, WB    Am Heart J 121 (1991): 951
16. Jardin, F    Int Care Med 29 (2003): 361
17. Zwissler, B    Der Anaesthesist 49 (2000): 788
18. Bhorade, S    Am J Respir    Crit Care Med 159 (1999): 571
19. Beuckelmann, DJ    Internist 38 (1997): 1020
20. Brent, B    Am J Cardiol 50 (1982): 255
21. Schulman, DS and RA Matthay    Cardiol Clin 10 (1992): 111
22. Vieillard-Baron, A    Crit Care Med 29 (2001): 1551
23. Brunet, F    Int Care Med 14 (1988): 474
24. Moore, TD    Am J Physiol Heart Circ Physiol 281 (2001): H2385–H2391
25. Atherton, JJ    Lancet 349 (1997): 1720
26. Kinch, JW    NEJM 330 (1994): 1211
27. Andersen, HR    JACC 10 (6) (1987): 1223
28. Isner, JM    Am J Cardiol 42 (1978): 885
29. Miro, AM    Heart-lung interaction. In: Tobin, MJ (ed) Principles and Practice of Mechanical Ventilation. McGraw-Hill, New York, 1994, pp 647–672
30. Vieillard-Baron, A    J Appl Physiol 87 (1999): 1664
31. Isobe, M    Am J Cardiol 59 (1987): 1245
32. Scharf, S    J Appl Physiol 49 (1980): 124
33. Parker, J    Crit Care Med 21 (1993): 131
34. Jardin, F    Catheter Cardiovasc Diag 16 (1989): 215
35. Jardin, F    Chest 99 (1991): 162
36. Jellinek, H    Crit Care Med 28 (2000): 672
37. Ganassini, A    Monaldi Arch Chest Dis 52 (1997): 68
38. Sessler, C    Crit Care Clin 14 (1998): 707
39. Pinsky, MR    Heart-lung interactions. In: Grenvik, A, Ayres, SM, Holbrook, PR and Shoemaker, WC (eds) Textbook of Critical Care, 4th edition. W. B. Saunders, Philadelphia, 2000, pp 1204–1221
40. Jardin, F    NEJM 304 (1981): 387
41. Viellard-Baron, A    Right ventricular function and positive pressure ventilation in clinical practice: From hemodynamic subsets to respirator settings. In: Pinsky, MR, Brochard, I. and Mancebo, J (eds) Applied Physiology in Intensive Care Medicine. Springer Verlag, Berlin, 2006, pp 207
42. Seige, M    Intensivmed 38 (2001): 299
43. Stoltzfus, DP    Anesthesiol Clin North Am 15 (1997): 797
44. Laver, MB    Crit Care Med 7 (1979): 509
45. Goldstein, JA    Circulation 65 (1982): 513

46. Hoeper, MM    Am J Respir Crit Care Med 165 (2002): 341

47. Ghio, S    JACC 37 (2001): 183

48. De Groote, P    JACC 32 (1998): 948

49. Redington, AN    Br Heart J 63 (1990): 45

50. Seki, S    Jpn J Thoracic Surg 28 (1977): 513

51. Magder, S    The cardiovascular Management of the Critically Ill Patient. In: Pinsky, MR (ed) Applied Cardiovascular Physiology. Springer-Verlag, Berlin, 1997, pp 28–35

52. Zapol, WM    NEJM 296 (1977): 476

53. Jardin, F    Chest 88 (1985): 653

54. Abraham, AS    Circ Res 24 (1969): 51

55. Simonneau, G    JACC 43 (2004): S 5

56. Willard, JEL    Cardiac catheterizations. In: Kloner, RA (ed) The Guide to Cardiology, 3rd edition. Greenwich, CT LeJacq Communicatioins, 1995, pp 151

57. Schmeck, J    Crit Care Med 26 (1998): 1868

58. Ware, LB    NEJM 342 (2000): 1334

59. Cheatham, ML    Crit Care Med 26 (1998): 1801

60. Vincent, JL    Perspectives in Crit Care 2 (1989): 141

61. Schulman, DS    Am J Med 84 (1988): 57

62. Sibbald, KJ    Crit Care Med 14 (1986): 852

63. Weitzenblum, E    Pulmonary hypertension due to chronic hypoxic lung disease. In: Peacock, AJ and Rubin LJ (eds) Pulmonary Circulation. Diseases and Their Treatment, 2nd edition. Oxford Press, New York, 2004, pp 376

64. Ishikawa, S J    Thorac Cardiovasc Surg 110 (1995): 271

65. Stewart, DJ    Ann Intern Med 114 (1991): 464

66. Kim, H    Eur Respir J 15 (2000): 640

67. Voelkel, NF    Circulation 114 (2006): 1883

68. Hassoun, P    34th congress of the SCCM, 15–19 Jan 2005, Phoenix, Arizona

69. Kerbaul, F    Crit Care Med 32 (2004): 1035

70. Kerbaul, F    Crit Care Med 34 (2006): 2814

71. Lee, FA    Cardiol Clin 10 (1992): 59

72. Chin, KM    Coron Artery Dis 16 (2005): 13

73. Pinsky, MR    Int Care Med 29 (2003): 19

74. Jardin, F    Ventricular interdependence: how does it impact on hemodynamic evaluation in clinical practice? In: Pinsky, MR, Brochard, L and Mancebo, J (eds) Applied Physiology in Intensive Care Medicine. Springer-Verlag, Berlin, 2006, pp 61

75. Kasper, W    Am Heart J 112 (1986): 1284

76. Matthay, RA    Chest 101 (1992): 255 S

77. Kosiborod, M    Semin Respir Crit Care 24 (2003): 245

78. Bristow, MR    Chest 114 (1998): 101 S

79. Wood, KE    Chest 121 (2002): 887

80. Shapiro, BP    Adv Pulmon Hypertens 5 (2006): 13

81. Mac Nee, W    BMJ 287 (1983): 1169

82. Bunnell, IL    Am J Med 39 (1968): 861

83. Dhainaut, JF    Int Care Med 14 (1988): 488

84. Schneider, AJ    Circ Shock 18 (1986): 53

85. Calvin, JE    Crit Care Med 9 (1981): 437

86. Rozich, JB   Circulation 86 (1992): 1718

87. Prewitt, RM and Ghignone   Crit Care Med 11 (1983): 346

88. Jardin, F   JACC 10 (1987): 1201

89. Hoffman, EA   Am J Physiol Heart Circ Physiol 249 (1985): H 883

90. Bleasdale, RA   Circulation 110 (2004): 2395

91. Madger, S   Curr Opin Crit Care 12 (2006): 219

92. Alzeer, A   Can J Anaesth 45 (1998): 798

93. Hamilton, DR   Circulation 90 (1994): 2492

94. Boltwood, CM   JACC 8 (1986): 1289

95. Smiseth, OA   JACC 27 (1996): 155

96. Darovic, GO   Hemodynamic Monitoring: Invasive and non-invasive Application, 2nd edition. W. B. Saunders Company, Philadelphia, 1995

97. Criley, JM and Ross, RS   Cardiovascular Physiology. Tarpon Springs, Florida, 1971

98. Tyberg, JV   Circulation 73 (1986): 428

99. Smiseth, OA   Am Heart J 108 (1983): 603–605

100. Traboulsi, M   Am Heart J 123 (1992): 1279

101. Belenkie, I   Circulation 80 (1989): 178

102. Belenkie, I   J Appl Physiol 96 (2004): 917–922

103. Smiseth, OA   Circulation 75 (1987): 1229

104. Badke, FR   Am J Physiol Heart Circ Physiol 242 (1982): H 611

105. Glantz, SA   Circ Res. 42 (1978): 433

106. Dell'Italia, LJ   J Appl Physiol 78 (1995): 2320

107. Belenkie, I   Circulation 78 (1988): 761

108. Jacobs, A   JACC 41 (2003): 1273

109. Ratliff, NB   Am J Cardiol 45 (1980): 217

110. Marving, J   Circulation 72 (1985): 502

111. Heywood, T   JACC 16 (1990): 611

112. Santamore, WP   J Appl Physiol 41 (1976): 362

113. Janicki, JS   Am J Physiol 238 (1980): H 494

114. Bemis, CE   Circ Res 34 (1974): 498

115. Williams, L and Frenneaux, M   Nature Clin Prac: Cardiovasc Med 3 (2006): 368–376

116. Belenkie, I   Ann Med 33 (2001): 236

117. Belenkie, I   Am Heart J 123 (1992): 733

118. Lee, JM   Circ Res 49 (1981): 533

119. Ishihara, T   Am J Cardiol 46 (1980): 744

120. Ross, J jr   Circulation 59 (1979): 32

121. Alderman, EL   Circulation 54 (1976): 667

122. Taylor, RR   Am J Physiol 218 (1967): 711

123. Kingma, I   Circulation 68 (1983): 1304

124. Jardin, F   Am Rev Resp Dis 129 (1984): 135

125. Mitchell, JP   Am Rev Respir Dis 145 (1992): 990

126. Metha, SR   JACC 37 (2001): 37

127. Frank, O   Z Biol 32 (1895): 3703 (English translation: Am Heart J 58 (1959): 282)

128. Starling, EH   The Linacre Lecture on the Law of the Heart. Longmans Green & Co, New York, 1918

129. Olsen, CO   Circ Res 52 (1983): 85

130. Molang, M    Circ Res 49 (1981): 52

131. Come, PC    JACC 10 (1987): 971

132. Slinker, BK    Am J Physiol 251 (1986): H 1062

133. Louie, EK    Circulation 92 (1995): 819

134. Galie`, N    JACC 41 (2003): 1380

135. Agostini, PG    Am J Cardiol 76 (1995): 793

136. Grant, DA    Am J Physiol 266 (1994): H 2327

137. Grant, DA    Circulation 94 (1996): 555

138. Kroecker, CA    Am J Physiol Heart Circ Physiol 284 (2003): H 2247

139. Applegate    Am J Physiol 262 (1992): H 1725

140. Flessas, AP and Ryan, TJ    Circulation 65 (1982): 1203

141. Rabkin, SW and Hsu, PH    Am J Physiol 229 (1975): 896

142. Braunwald, E    Heart Diseases. E. Saunders and Co, Philadelphia, 1984, pp 1573

143. Calvin, JE    Circulation 84 (1991): 852

144. Goldstein, JA    Circulation 82 (1990): 359

145. Vieillard-Baron, A    Am J Respir Crit Care Med 168 (2003): 1270

146. Kimichi, A    JACC 4 (1984): 945

147. Parker, MM    Chest 97 (1990): 126

148. Sagie, A    JACC 24 (1994): 446

149. Nath, J    JACC 43 (2004): 405

150. Feneley, MP    Circ Res 65 (1989): 135

151. Stein, PD    Am J Cardiol 44 (1979): 1050

152. Calvin, JE    J Crit Care 4 (1989): 251

153. Calvin, JE    Am J Physiol 20 (1986): H 722

154. Starr, I    Am Heart J 26 (1943): 291

155. Bellamy, RF    Am J Physiol 238 (1980): H 481

156. Farb, A    Cardiol Clin 10 (1992): 1

157. Torbicke, A    Circulation 108 (2003): 844

158. Vlahakes, GJ    Circulation 63 (1981): 87

159. Brooks, H    J Clin Invest 50 (1971): 2176

160. Mebazaa, A    Acute right ventricular failure – from pathophysiology to new treatments. In: Pinsky, MR, Brochard, L and Mancebo, J (eds) Applied Physiology in Intensive Care Medicine. Springer-Verlag, Berlin, 2006, pp 217

161. Urabe, Y    Circ Res 57 (1985): 96

162. Gold, FL    Circ Res 51 (1982): 204

163. Sibbald, WJ    Crit Care Med 11 (1983): 339

164. Goldstein, JA    Progress in Cardiovasc. Dis 49 (1998): 325

165. Molaug, M    Acta Physiol Scand 116 (1982): 245

166. Zwissler, B    Europ J Med Res 3 (1999): 231

167. Goldstein, JA    JACC 16 (1990): 181

168. Goldstein, JA    JACC 19 (1992): 704

169. Armour, JA    Cardiology 58 (1973): 65

170. Santamore, WP    Ann Thorac Surg 61 (1996): 350

171. Klima, UP    Ann Thorac Cardiovasc surg 5 (1999): 74

172. Gehlbach, BK    Chest 125 (2004): 669

173. Ravenscraft, SA    Chest 103 (1993): 54

174. Dimopoulow, I    Respir Med 92 (1998): 1321

175. Cournaund, A    Am J Physiol 152 (1948): 162

176. Pinsky, MR    Curr Opin Crit Care 8 (2002): 26

177. Klinger, JR    Crit Care Clin 12 (1996): 841

178. Artucio, H    Int Care Med 23 (1997): 836

179. Brienza, N    Int Care Med 32 (2006): 267

180. Jardin, F    Crit Care Med 13 (1985): 952

181. Jardin, F    Anesthesiology 72 (1990): 966

182. Morgan, B    Circ Res 26 (1965): 493

183. Fessler, H    Am Rev Respir Dis 146 (1992): 4

184. Schmitt, JM    Crit Care Med 29 (2000): 1154

185. Vieillard-Baron, A    Am J Respir Crit Care Med 165 (2002): 1107

186. Suter, P    NEJM 292 (1975): 284

187. Robotham, JL    Cardiorespiratory interactions. In: Bone, RC (ed) Pulmonary and Critical Care Medicine. Volume 2, section 14, Mosby-Year Book Inc., St Louis, 1993, pp 1–25

188. Permutt, S    Anesthesiology 69 (1988): 157

189. Peters, J    Am J Appl Physiol 257 (1989): H 120

190. Armaganidis, A    Intensivmed 34 (1997): 696

191. Schulman, DS    Am J Med 84 (1988): 57

192. Calvin, JE    J Cardiothoracic and Vascular Anesthesia 5 (1991): 507

193. Mac Nee, W    Am J Respir Crit Care Med 150 (1994): 833

194. Richens, JM    Clin Sci 62 (1982): 255

195. Leuchte, HH    JACC 43 (2004): 764

196. Nagaya, N    JACC 31 (1998): 202

197. Kruger, S    Am Heart J 147 (2004): 60

198. Pruszcczyk, P    Europ Respir J 22 (2003): 649

199. Tulevski, II    Thromb Haemost 86 (2001): 1193

200. Kucher, N    Circulation 107 (2003): 2545

201. Logeart, D    Int Care Med 33 (2007): 286

202. Nagaya, N    Circulation 102 (2000): 865

203. Tulevski, II    Heart 86 (2001): 27

204. Remme, WJ    Eur Heart J 22 (2001): 1527

205. Heart Fail Soc of America (HFSA) practice guidelines    J Card Fail 5 (1999): 357

206. Kucher, N    Europ Heart J 24 (2003): 1651

207. Kucher, N    Circulation 107 (2003): 1576

208. Konstantinidis, S    Circulation 106 (2002): 1263

209. The GUSTO-Investigators    NEJM 329 (1993): 673

210. Eddy, AL    J Crit Care 4 (1989): 58

211. Jardin, F    Chest 88 (1985): 34

212. Michaux, I    Right ventricle. In: Poelaert, J and Skarvan, K (eds) Transaesophageal Echocardiography in Anaesthesia and Intensive Care Medicine, 2nd edition. BMJ Books, 2004, Chapter 8, pp 145

213. Poelaert, J    Hemodynamics. In: Poelaert, J and Skarvan, K (eds) Transaesophageal Echocardiography in Anaesthesia and Intensive Care Medicine, 2nd edition. BMJ Books, 2004, Chapter 10, pp 176

214. Goldhaber, SZ    Ann Intern Med 136 (2002): 691

215. Jardin, F    Chest 111 (1997): 209

216. Lualdi, JC    Am Heart J 130 (1995): 1276

217. Ribeiro, A    Am Heart J 135 (1998): 868
218. Mansencal, N    Am J Cadiol 95 (2005): 1260
219. Kostrubiec, M    Europ Heart J 26 (2005): 2166
220. McConnell, MV    Am J Cardiol 78 (1996): 469
221. Forfia, P    Am J Respir Crit Care Med 174 (2006): 1034
222. Kaul, S    Am Heart J 107 (1984): 526
223. Karatasakis, GT    Am J Cardiol 82 (1998): 329
224. Ghio, S    Am J Cardiol 85 (2000): 837
225. Samad, BA    Am J Cardiol 90 (2002): 778
226. Hebert, JL    Am J Cardiol 93 (2004): 728
227. Shah, AR    Echocardiography 17 (2000): 513
228. Urheim, S    Am J Cardiol 96 (2005): 1173
229. Leschke, M    Der Internist 48 (2007): 948
230. Florea, VG    Chest 118 (2000): 1063
231. Hatle, L and Sutherland, G    Echokardiographie Update. 2nd and 3rd Dec. 2005, München/Germany
232. Ueti, OM    Heart 88 (2002): 244
233. Gan, TJ    Am J Physiol Heart Circ Physiol 290 (2006): H 1528
234. Kasper, W    Br Heart J 70 (1993): 352
235. Pinsky, M    Int Care Med 26 (2000): 1164
236. York, PG    Circulation 70 (1984): 657
237. Ihlen, H    Br. Heart J 51 (1984): 54
238. Berger, M    JACC 6 (1985): 359
239. Hatle, L    Br Heart J 45 (1981): 157
240. Abbas, AE    JACC 41 (2003): 1021
241. Grossman, W    Cardiac Catheterization, Angiography and Intervention, 6th edition. p 172, table 8.1
242. Zwissler, B    Intensivmed 38 (2001): 264
243. Chen, P    Circulation 97 (1998): 1606
244. Louie, EK    Circulation 92 (1995): 819
245. Ghignone, M    Anesthesiology 60 (1984): 132
246. Goldstein, JA    JACC 2 (1983): 270
247. Dell'Italia, LJ    Circulation 72 (1985): 1327
248. Love, JC    Am Heart J 108 (1984): 5
249. Menon, V    Heart 88 (2002): 531
250. Hirsch, LJ    Chest 95 (1989): 1333
251. Ducas, JM    Am Rev Respir Dis 146 (1992): 307
252. Morelli, A    Crit Care Med 34 (2006): 2287
253. Braat, SH    Am Heart J 113 (1987): 257
254. Bowers, TR    NEJM 338 (1998): 933
255. Schuler, G    Am J Cardiol 54 (1984): 951
256. Hochman, JS    JAMA 285 (2001): 190
257. Popatov, EV    J Heart Lung Transplant 20 (2001): 918
258. Goldhaber, SZ    Lancet 353 (1999): 1386
259. Goldhaber, SZ    Circulation 108 (2003): 2834
260. Figulla, R    34th Crit Care Congress in Phoenix, Arizona, 15 to 19 June 2005
261. Konstantinidis, A    NEJM 347 (2002): 1143
262. Kucher, N    Ann Intern Med 165 (2005): 1777

263. Grifoni, S    Circulation 101 (2000): 2817
264. Kasper, W    Heart 77 (1997): 346
265. Robinson, GV    BMJ 332 (2006): 156
266. Kiil, J    Acta Chirurgica Scand 144 (1978): 427
267. Arcasoy, SM    Chest 115 (1999): 1695
268. Franke, I    Intensivmed. 41 (2004): 192
269. Tai, NRM    British J of Surgery 86 (1999): 853
270. Kucher, N    Europ Heart J 24 (2003): 366
271. Riedel, M    Heart 85 (2001): 351
272. Konstantinidis, A    Circulation 96 (1997): 882
273. Stevenson, BG    Europ Heart J 28 (2007): 2517
274. Gold, FL    Circ Res 51 (1982): 196
275. Cuenoud, HF    Am J Pathol 92 (1978): 421
276. Watts, JA    J Mol Cell Cardiol 41 (2006): 296
277. Steiner, S    Internist 45 (2004): 1101
278. Mercat, A    Crit Care Med 27 (1999): 540
279. Pinsky, MR    J Crit Care 11 (1996): 95
280. Vincent, J-L and Weil, MH    Crit Care Med 34 (2006): 1333
281. Michard, F    Chest 124 (2003): 1900
282. Kirov, MY    Crit Care 8 (2004): R 451
283. Menon, V    JACC 36 (2000): 1071
284. Dellinger, RP    Crit Care Med 32 (2004): 858
285. Michard, F    Am J Respir Crit Care Med 162 (2000): 134
286. Sakr, Y    Crit Care Med 34 (2006): 589
287. Levy, MM    Crit Care Med 33 (2005): 2194
288. Martin, C    Intensivmed 37 (2000): 507
289. Eckstein, J    Am Heart J 63 (1962): 119
290. Molloy, WD    Am Rev Respir Dis 130 (1984): 870
291. DiGiantomasso, D    Int Care Med 28 (2002): 1804
292. Müllner, M    Cochrane Database Syst Rev 2004, issue 3, Art No: CD 003709. DOI: 10.1002/14651858.CD003709. pub2; and: http://www.cochrane.org/review/en/ab003709.html
293. Martin, C    Crit Care Med 28 (2000): 2758
294. Hochman, JS    NEJM 341 (1999): 625
295. AHA/ACC guidelines    Circulation 100 (1999): 1016
296. Williams, JF    Circulation 92 (1995): 2764
297. Halperin, HR    Circulation 73 (1986): 539
298. Cheatham, ML    Int J Crit Care Autum (2000): 1–6
299. Torum, M    Congress of the Dep. Cardiology, University of Indonesia, 29. Sep. 2005
300. Nico, HJ    Circulation 92 (1995): 3183
301. Bourdarias, JP    Europ Heart J 16 (suppl I) (1995): 2
302. Ballester, E    Am Rev Respir Dis 141 (1990): 558
303. Anzueta, A    Acute Exacerbation of Chronic Obstructive Pulmonary Diseases: What are the impact of broncho-dilators, corticosteroids and antibiotics. In: Esteban, A, Anzueto, A and Cook, DJ (eds) Evidence-Based Management of Patients with Respiratory Failure. Springer Verlag, Berlin – New York – Heidelberg, 2004, pp 79
304. ATS/ ERS guidelines 2004 and updated September 8th 2005. http://www.thoracic.org./go/copd

305. Matthey, RA    Clin Chest Med 4 (1983): 269

306. Ferlinz, J    Prog Cardiovasc Dis25 (1982): 225

307. Barr, RG    BMJ 327 (2003): 643

308. Mahon, JL    Chest 115 (1999): 38

309. Sydow, M    Int Care Med 19 (1993): 467

310. Packer, MM    Ann Intern Med 103 (1985): 258

311. Ghofrani, HA    Lancet 360 (2002): 895

312. Gatecel, C    Anesthesiology 82 (1995): 588

313. Langer, F    Europ J Anaesthesiol 18 (2001): 770

314. Haraldsson, A    J Cardiothorac Vasc Anesth 10 (1996): 864

315. Mosquera, I    Transplant Proc. 34 (2002): 166

316. Olschewski, H    Am J Respir Crit Care Med 160 (1999): 600

317. Olschewski, H    Intensive Care Med 24 (1998): 631

318. Hoeper, MM    NEJM 342 (2000): 1866

319. Walmrath, D    Intensivmed 34 (1997): 370

320. Bone, RC    Chest 96 (1989): 114

321. Lowson, SM    Crit Care Med 30 (2002): 2762

322. Lowson, SM    Anesthesiology 96 (2002): 1504

323. Zwissler, B    J Anästh Intensivbehandlung 5 (1999): 224

324. Christenson, J    Am J Respir Crit Care Med 161 (2000): 1443

325. Bhatia, S    Mayo Clin Proc 78 (2003): 1207

326. Michelakis, E    Circulation105 (2002): 2398

327. Lepore, JJ    Am J Cardiol 90 (2002): 677

328. Krowka, MJ    Liver Transplantation 10 (2004): 174

329. Rafanan, AL    Chest 188 (2000): 1497

330. Zamanian, RT    Crit Care Med 35 (2007): 2037

331. O'Connor, CM    Am Heart J 138 (1999): 78

332. Packer, MM    NEJM 352 (1991): 1468

333. Löllgen, H and Drexler, H    Crit Care Med 18 (suppl) (1990): S 61

334. Vincent, JL    Crit Care Med 16 (1988): 659

335. Leier, CV    Prog. Cardiovasc Dis 41 (1998): 207

336. Holtz, J    Intensivmed. 37 (2000): 644

337. Burger, AJ    Am Heart J 144 (2002): 1102

338. Ewy, GA    JACC 33 (1999): 572

339. Cuffe, MS    JAMA 287 (2002): 1541

340. Abraham, WT    J Card Fail 9 (suppl 1) (2003): S 81

341. Yokoshiki, H    Europ J Pharmacol 333 (1997): 249

342. De Witt, BJ    Anesth Analg 94 (2002): 1427

343. Slawsky, MT    Circulation 102 (2000): 2222

344. Leather, HA    Crit Care Med 31 (2003): 2339

345. Innes, CA    Drugs 63 (2003): 2651

346. Haikala, H    J Cardiovasc Pharmacol 25 (1995): 794

347. Sonntag, S    JACC 43 (2004): 2177

348. Haikala, H    Idrug 3 (2000): 1199

349. Delle Karth, G    Wien Klin Wochenschr 116 (2004): 6

350. Hermann, H-P    Intensivmed 41 (2004): 451

351.  Rabuel, C and Mebazaa, A    Int Care Med 32 (2006): 799

352.  Boehmer, JP    Crit Care Med 34 (Suppl) (2006): S 268

353.  Anderson, RD    JACC 30 (1997): 708

354.  Bur, A    Rescuciation 53 (2002): 259

355.  Martin, C    Chest 103 (1993): 1826

356.  Kiely, DG    Chest 109 (1996): 1215

357.  Rose, CE    Circ Res 52 (1982): 76

358.  Fullerton, DA    Am Thorac Surg 61 (1996): 696

359.  Viitanen, A    Anaesthsiology 73 (1990): 393

360.  Morray, JP    Paediatr 113 (1988): 474

361.  Roberts, DH    Chest 120 (2001): 1547

362.  Flenley, DC    Clin Chest Med. 4 (1983): 297

363.  Timms, RM    Ann Intern Med 102 (1985): 29

364.  McFadden, ER and Braunwald, E    Cor pulmonale and pulmonary embolism. In: Braunwald (ed) Textbook of Cardiovasc. Medicine. W. B. Saunders Company, Philadelphia, 1984

365.  Seki, S    Jpn J Thoraci Surg 28 (1977): 513

366.  Isner, JM    Am Heart J 102 (1981): 792

367.  Topol, EJ    Ann Intern Med 96 (1982): 594

368.  Calvin, JE    Circ Res 56 (1985): 40

369.  Mebazaa, A    Meeting of the Acute Cardiac Care Group of the ESC in Prague, 21st to 24th Oct 2006, during the session "Do we care enough for the RV in the ICU?"

370.  Groeneveld, AJ    J Appl Physiol 89 (2000): 89

371.  Nicod, LP    Swiss Med WKLY 133 (2003): 103

372.  Brijker, F    Chest 121 (2002): 377

373.  Heinemann, HO    Am J Med 64 (1978): 367

374.  Sylvester, JT    Clin Chest Med 4 (1983): 111

375.  Fuster, V    Circulation 70 (1984): 580

376.  Rich, S    NEJM 327 (1992): 76

377.  Welsh, H    Chest 110 (1996): 710

378.  Thompson, BT    Am J Respir Crit Care Med 149 (1994): 1512

379.  Spence, CR    Am Rev Respir Dis 148 (1993): 241

380.  Mathur, PN    Ann Intern Med 95 (1981): 283

381.  Jezek, V    Br Heart J 35 (1973): 2

382.  Sibbald, WJ    Chest 73 (1978): 583

383.  Morrissey, B    Crit Care Med 33 (2005): 691

384.  Moloney, ED    Eur Respir J 21 (2003): 720

385.  Dorfmuller, P    Eur Respir J 22 (2003): 358

386.  Post, F    Intensivmed 43 (2006): 636

387.  Brown, KA    JACC 3 (1984): 895

388.  Haddad, E    Anesthesiology 92 (2000): 1821

# Chapter 5

1.  Paulus, WJ    European Heart Journal 28 (2007): 2539

2.  Vasan, RS    Circulation 101 (2000): 2118

3. Angeja, BG    Circulation 107 (2003): 659
4. Mauer, MS    JACC 44 (2004): 1543
5. Zile, MR    Circulation 105 (2002): 1387
6. Burkhoff, D    Circulation 107 (2003): 656
7. Oh, JK    JACC 47 (2006): 500
8. Zile, MR    JACC 41 (2003): 1519
9. Ghandi, SK    NEJM 344 (2001): 17
10. Grossman, W    Circulation 81 (suppl III) (1990): III-1
11. Kitzman, DW    JAMA 288 (2002): 2144
12. Zile, MR    NEJM 350 (2004): 1953
13. Kitzman, DW    JACC 17 (1991): 1065
14. Hadano, Y    Am J Cardiol 97 (2006): 1025
15. Skaluba, SJ    Circulation 109 (2004): 972
16. Yu, C-M    Circulation 105 (2002): 1195
17. Xie, GY    JACC 24 (1994): 132
18. van Heerebeek, L    Circulation 113 (2006): 1966
19. Hoit, BD    Crit Care Med 35 (2007): S 340
20. Grossman, W    Circulation 101 (2000): 2020
21. Banerjee, P    JACC 39 (2002): 138
22. Vasan, RS    JACC 33 (1999): 1948
23. Kupari, M    J Intern Med 241 (1997): 387
24. Owan, TE    NEJM 355 (2006): 251
25. Abhayaratna, WP    Heart 92 (2006): 1259
26. Steendijk, P    Cardiovasc Res 64 (2004): 9
27. Vasan, RS    JACC 26 (1995): 1565
28. Thomas, MD    Eur J Heart Fail 6 (2004): 125
29. Cleland, JG    Eur Heart J 24 (2003): 442
30. Owan, TE    Prog Cardiovasc Dis 47 (2005): 320
31. Yancy, CW    JACC 47 (2006): 76
32. Liao, L    Arch Intern Med 166 (2006): 112
33. Bhatia, RS    NEJM 355 (2006): 260
34. Zile, MR    Circulation 105 (2002): 1503
35. Gottdiener, JS    JACC 35 (2000): 1628
36. Klapholz, M    Circulation 104 (suppl II) (2001): II-689
37. Appleton, CP    JACC 22 (1993): 1972
38. Dumesnil, JG    J Am Soc Echocardiogr 15 (2002): 1226
39. Devereux, RB    Am J Cardiol 86 (2000): 1090
40. Maurer, MS    J Car Fail 11 (2005): 177
41. Avolio, AP    Circulation 71 (1985): 202
42. Hundley, WG    JACC 38 (2001): 796
43. Chen, C-H    JACC 32 (1998): 1221
44. Grossman, W    NEJM 325 (1991): 1557
45. Boudina, S    Circulation 115 (2007): 3213
46. Munagata, VK    Circulation 111 (2005): 1128
47. Kawaguchi, M    Circulation 107 (2003): 714
48. Schwartzkopff, B    Der Internist 41 (2000): 253

49. Pak, PH    Circulation 94 (1996): 52
50. Borbely, A    Circulation 111 (2005): 774
51. Makarenko, I    Circ Res 95 (2004): 708
52. Nagueh, SF    Circulation 110 (2004): 155
53. Neagoe, C    Circulation 106 (2002): 1333
54. Ahmed, SH    Criculation 113 (2006): 2089
55. Heymans, S    Circulation 112 (2005): 1136
56. Spinale, FG    Circulation 102 (2000): 1944
57. Baicu, CF    Circulation 111 (2005): 2306
58. Gaasch, WH    Ann Rev Med 55 (2004): 373
59. Urheim, S    J Am Soc Echocardiogr 15 (2002): 225
60. Westerhof, N, Stergiopulos, N and Noble, M    Snapshots of Hemodynamics. Chapter 11: Compliance. Springer Science and Business Media, Boston, 2005, pp 41
61. Hatle, L    Eur Heart Journal 28 (2007): 2421
62. Strauer, BE    Hypertension 6 (6 Pt 2) (1984): III 4
63. Strauer, BE    J Hypertens 16 (1996): 1221
64. Pickering, TG    J Clin Hypertens 6 (2004): 647
65. Caruana, L    BMJ 321 (2000): 215
66. Wilson, JR    Circulation 92 (1995): 47
67. Yellin, EL    Prog Cardiovasc Dis 32 (1990): 247
68. Leite-Moreira, AF    Cardiovasc Res 43 (1999): 344
69. Najjer, SS    JACC 44 (2004): 611
70. Gibson, DG    Br Heart J 36 (1974): 1066
71. Iriarte, M    Am J Cardiol 71 (1993): 308
72. Cotter, G    Europ J Heart Fail 5 (2003): 443
73. Ware, LB    NEJM 353 (2005): 2788
74. Straub, NC    Physiol Rev 54 (1974): 678
75. Borlaug, BA    Trends Cardiovasc Med 16 (2006): 273
76. Litwin, SE    JACC 22 (1993): 49 A
77. De Mots, H    Pulmonary Oedema. In: Cardiac Emergencies. Williams and Wilkins Company, Baltimore, 1978, pp 173–223
78. Brutsaert, DL    Physiol Rev 69 (1989): 1228
79. Leite-Moreira, AF    Circulation 90 (1994): 2481
80. Gaasch, WH    Am J Physiol 239 (1980): H 1
81. Kass, DA    Circ Res 94 (2004): 1533
82. Leite-Moreira, AF    Am J Physiol Heart Circ Physiol 280 (2001): H 51
83. Gillebert, TC    Heart Fail Rev 5 (2000): 345
84. Little, WC    Heart Fail Rev 5 (2000): 300
85. Shah, PM    Curr Probl Cardiol 17 (1992): 783
86. Schannwell, CM    Der Internist 48 (2007): 909
87. Burnett, JC    Science 231 (1986): 1145
88. Rodehetter, RJ    JACC 44 (2004): 740
89. Yamanaka, T    Am Heart J 152 (2006): 966e 1–7
90. Vinereanu, D    Heart 89 (2003): 449
91. Warner, JG    JACC 33 (1999): 1567
92. Aroesky, JM    Circulation 71 (1985): 889

93.  Watanabe, J    Circulation 88 (1993): 2929

94.  Stern, S    Circulation 106 (2002): 1906

95.  Kelly, PR    Circ Res 71 (1992): 490

96.  Kass, DA    Ann Biomed Eng 20 (1992): 41

97.  Sunagawa, K    Am J Physiol 245 (1983): H773

98.  Kass, DA    Heart Fail Rev 7 (2002): 51

99.  Saba, PS    J Hypertens 13 (1995): 971

100.  Liu, CP    Circulation 88 (1993): 1893

101.  Starling, MR    Am Heart J 125 (1993): 1659

102.  Asanoi, H    Circ Res 65 (1989): 483

103.  Courtois, M    Circulation 85 (1992): 1132

104.  Dent, JM    Am J Physiol 269 (1995): H 2100

105.  Nichols, WW et al.    In: McDonald's Blood Flow in Arteries: Theoretical, Experimental and Clinical Principles, 4th edition. Arnold, London, 1997

106.  Brutsaert, DL    JACC 22 (1993): 318

107.  Sanderson, JE    Heart 89 (2003): 1281

108.  Yu, CM    Am Heart J 134 (1997): 426

109.  Bellot, JF    Causes and onset of pulmonary oedema. Acute Cardiac Care Congress 21st to 24th Oct 2006, Prague, reference 635

110.  Little, WC    Hypertensive pulmonary oedema. Acute Cardiac Care Congress 21st to 24th Oct 2006, Prague, reference 636

111.  Kitzman, DW    Am J Cardiol 87 (2001): 413

112.  Klapholz, M    JACC 43 (2004): 1432

113.  Senni, M    Circulation 98 (1998): 2282

114.  Redfield, MM    JAMA 289 (2003): 194

115.  Mirsky, J    Circulation 69 (1989): 836

116.  Kass, DA    Cardiol Clin 18 (2000): 57

117.  Wang, TJ    Ann Intern Med 138 (2003): 907

118.  Hogg, K    JACC 43 (2004): 317

119.  Jensen, J    J Am Soc Echocardiogr 10 (1997): 60

120.  Gaasch, WH    JAMA 271 (1994): 1276

121.  European Study Group on Diastolic Heart Failure    Eur Heart J 19 (1998): 990

122.  Yturralde, RF    Prog Cardiovasc Dis 47 (2005): 314

123.  Nagueh, SF    Circulation 98 (1998): 1644

124.  McCullagh, WH    Circulation 45 (1975): 943

125.  Westerhof, N; Stergiopulos, N and Noble, M    Snapshots of Hemodynamics. Springer Science and Business Media, Boston, 2005, Chapter 11, p 45

126.  Braunwald, E    Heart Diseases, 5th edtion. 1997, p 403

127.  Zile, MR    Mod. Concepts Cardiovasc. Dis 59 (1990): 1

128.  Tyberg, JV    Circulation 66 (1979): 461

129.  Little, WC    Prog. Cardiovasc Dis 32 (1996): 273

130.  Carabello, BA    Circulation 105 (2002): 2701

131.  Solomon, SD    Circulation 112 (2005): 3738

132.  Lang, RM    Eur J Echocardiography 7 (2006): 79

133.  Zile, MR    Circulation 104 (2001): 779

134.  He, KL    Cardiovasc Res 64 (2004): 72

135. Petrie, MC    Heart 87 (2002): 29

136. Mahler, F    Am J Cardiol 35 (1975): 625

137. Ross, J jr    Prog Cardiovasc Dis 18 (1976): 255

138. Borrow, KM    JACC 20 (1992): 787

139. Kreulen, TH    Circulation 51 (1975): 677

140. Gunther, S    Circulation 59 (1979): 679

141. Carabello, BA    Circulation 64 (1981): 1212

142. Zile, MR    JACC 3 (1984): 235

143. DeSimone, G    J Hypertens 17 (1999): 1001

144. Vinereanu, D    Am J Cardiol 8 (2001): 53

145. Takeda, S    Heart 86 (2001): 52

146. Hasegawa, H    JACC 41 (2003): 1590

147. Lundbäck, S    Acta Physiol Scand 55 (suppl) (1986): 1

148. Högelund, C    Acta Med Scand 224 (1988): 557

149. Henein, MY    Heart 81 (1999): 229

150. Yip, G    Heart 87 (2002): 1219

151. Schiller, NB    Circulation 84 (suppl 3) (1991): 1280

152. Issaz, K    J Am Soc Echo 6 (1993): 166

153. Pai, A    Am J Cardiol 67 (1991): 222

154. Alam, M    J Am Soc Echocardiogr 5 (1992): 427

155. Willenheimer, R    Heart 78 (1997): 230

156. Hoglund, C    J Intern Med 226 (1989): 251

157. Hatle, L and Sutherland, G    Echokardiographie update, München Dec. 2005

158. Alam, M    Europ Heart J 13 (1992): 194

159. Alam, M    Am J Cardiol 69 (1992): 565

160. Krandis, A    Europ J of Heart Fail 3 (2001): 147

161. Willenheimer, R    Coron Artery Dis 8 (1997): 719

162. Wiggers, CJ    Am J Physiol 56 (1921): 415

163. Ohte, N    Am J Cardiol 82 (1998): 1414

164. Oki, T    Am J Cardiol 79 (1997): 921

165. Upton, MT    Br Heart J 38 (1976): 1001

166. Kitabatake, A    Jpn Circ J 46 (1982): 92

167. Gibson, DG    Heart 89 (2003): 231

168. Lim, T    Eur J Heart Fail 8 (2006): 38

169. Caruana, L    Eur Heart J 20 (1999): 393

170. Thomas, MD    Heart 92 (2006): 603

171. Cahill, JM    Eur J Heart Fail 4 (2002): 473

172. Palmieri, V    J Am Soc Echocardiogr 18 (2005): 99

173. Giannuzzi, P    JACC 23 (1994): 1630

174. Nishimura, R    JACC 30 (1997): 8

175. Rossvoll, O    JACC 21 (1993): 1687

176. Rocca, HP    J Am Soc Echocardiogr 13 (2000): 599

178. Hadano, Y    Circ J 69 (2005): 432

179. Yamamoto, K    J Am Soc Echocardiogr 10 (1997): 52

180. Sohn, D    JACC 30 (1997): 474

181. Nagueh, S    JACC 31 (2001): 278

182. Ha, J    J Am Soc Echocardiogr 18 (2005): 63

183. Poelaert, J    Anaesthesia 53 (1998): 55

184. Ommen, S    Circulation 102 (2000): 1788

185. Nagueh, S    JACC 30 (1997): 1527

186. Nagueh, S    Circulation 98 (1998): 1644

187. Gonzales-Vilchez, F    J Am Soc Echocardiogr 15 (2002): 1245

188. Olson, JJ    J Am Soc Echocardiogr 19 (2006): 83

189. Calvin, JE    Crit Care Med 9 (1981): 437

190. Cheatham, ML    Crit Care Med 26 (1998): 1801

191. Culle, DJ    Crit Care Med 17 (1989): 118

192. Pritchett, AM    JACC 45 (2005): 87

193. Paulus, WJ    Circulation 86 (1992): 1175

194. Yamakado, T    Circulation 95 (1997): 917

195. Little, WC    Prog Cardiovasc Dis 32 (1990): 273

196. Watanabe, S    Eur Heart J 26 (2005): 2277

197. Tschope, C    Eur Heart J 27 (2006): 832

198. Ando, T    Chest 110 (1996): 462

199. Tulevskill, HA    Thromb Haemost 86 (2001): 1193

200. Thorens, JB    Eur Respir J 10 (1997): 2553

201. Redfield, MM    Circulation 109 (2004): 3176

202. Maisel, AS    JACC 41 (2003): 2010

203. Hoppe, UC    Der Internist 48 (2007): 929

204. Fonarow, GC    Rev Cardiovasc Med 3 (suppl 4) (2002): S 18

205. Mehra, M    Am Heart J 151 (2006): 571

206. Northbridge, D    Lancet 47 (1996): 667

207. Gheorghiade, M    Europ Heart J Supplements 7 (Supplement B) (2007): B 13

208. Nussbacher, A    Am J Physiol 277 (1999): H 1863

209. Everly, MJ    Ann Pharmacother 38 (2004): 286

210. Chobanian, AV    JAMA 289 (2003): 2560

211. Yu, CM    Pacing Clin Electrphysiol 24 (2001): 979

212. Friedrich, SP    Circulation 90 (1994): 2761

213. Schunkert, H    Circulation 87 (1993): 1328

214. Diez, J    Circulation 105 (2002): 2512

215. Warner, JG jr    JACC 33 (1999): 1567

216. Dahlhof, B    Lancet 359 (2002): 995

217. Yusuf, S    Lancet 362 (2003): 777

218. Carson, P    JACC 27 (1996): 642

219. Eriksson, SV    Cardiology 85 (1994): 137

220. The Digitalis Investigation Group    NEJM 336 (1997): 525

# Index

# Abbreviations

| | |
|---|---|
| ACS | Acute coronary syndrome |
| AMI | Acute myocardial infarction |
| ARDS | Acute respiratory distress syndrome |
| BP | Blood pressure |
| CF | Cardiac function |
| CI | Cardiac index |
| CO | Cardiac output |
| CPI | Cardiac power index |
| CPO | Cardiac power output |
| CPP | Coronary perfusion pressure |
| CS | Cardiogenic shock |
| CVP | Central venous pressure |
| dp/dt | Change in (left) ventricular pressure per time |
| DVI | Diastolic ventricular interaction |
| $E_a$ | Effective arterial elastance |
| $E_{es}$ | Endsystolic chamber elastance |
| EF | Ejection fraction (left ventricular); RV-EF (ejection fraction right ventricle) |
| E.O. hypo | End-organ hypoperfusion |
| ESV | Endsystolic volume |
| EVLW(I) | Extra vascular lung water (index) |
| GEDV | Global end diastolic volume |
| HF | Heart failure |
| HFNEF | Heart failure with normal EF |
| HFREF | Heart failure with reduced EF |
| HR | Heart rate |
| ICP | Intracerebral pressure |
| IHD | Ischaemic heart disease |
| ITBV(I) | Intra thoracic blood volume (index) |
| LV | Left ventricle |
| LVEDA | Left ventricular end-diastolic area |
| LVEDD | Left ventricular end-diastolic diameter |
| LVEDP | Left ventricular end diastolic pressure; also called intracavitary LVEDP |
| LVESP | End-systolic left ventricular pressure |
| LVESV | End-systolic left ventricular volume |
| LV-H | Left ventricular hypertrophy |
| LVOT | Left ventricular outflow tract |
| MAP | Mean arterial (blood) pressure |
| MR | Mitral valve regurgitation |
| PBV | Pulmonary blood volume |
| PCWP | Pulmonary capillary wedge pressure |

| | |
|---|---|
| PE | Pulmonary embolism |
| PEEP | Positive end-expiratory pressure |
| PH | Pulmonary hypertension |
| PLR | Passive leg raising |
| PP | Pericardial pressure |
| PP-V | Pulse pressure variation |
| P-V diagram | Pressure-volume diagram of the ventricle cycle |
| PVPI | Pulmonary venous permeability index |
| RA | Right atrium |
| RAP | Right atrial pressure |
| RCA | Right coronary artery |
| RV | Right ventricle |
| RV-AMI | Acute myocardial infarction of the right ventricle |
| RVEDP | Right ventricular end diastolic pressure |
| RVEDV | Right ventricular end diastolic volume |
| sBP | Systolic blood pressure |
| $ScvO_2$ | Central venous oxygen saturation (central vein, i.e. vena cava inferior) |
| SP-V | Systolic pressure variation |
| SV(I) | Stroke volume (index) |
| $SvO_2$ | Mixed venous oxygen saturation (pulmonary artery) |
| SVR(I) | Systemic vascular resistance (index) |
| SV-V | Stroke volume variation |
| SW(I) | Stroke work (index) |
| UO | Urinary output |
| VT | Ventricular tachycardia |